STEP TRAINING PLUS
❖ THE WAY TO FITNESS ❖

Karen S. Mazzeo, M.Ed.
Bowling Green State University

Lauren M. Mangili, M.Ed.
Bowling Green State University

Morton Publishing Company
925 West Kenyon Avenue, Unit 12
Englewood, Colorado 80110

Typography by Ash Street Typecrafters, Inc., Denver, Colorado
Cover Design by Bob Schram, Bookends, Inc., Boulder, Colorado
Illustrations by Susan Strawn, Loveland, Colorado
Edited by Carolyn Acheson, Riverbank, California
Cover Photo and Interior Photography by Jeffrey Hall Photography, Haskins, Ohio

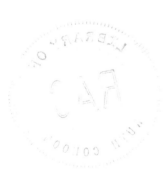

Printed in the United States of America

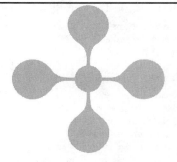

TABLE OF CONTENTS

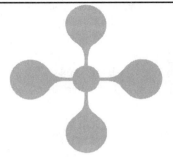

INTRODUCTION

Bench/step training, or step training, is the hottest aerobic trend of this decade, sweeping the aerobics fitness industry with a new burst of enthusiasm. Step training, which uses a 4-12" step bench, is a safe and efficient method of achieving and maintaining physical fitness. Even though it is a relatively new activity, it rapidly is attaining the unique distinction as *the* way to fitness in the 1990s.

Step-Training Plus ÷ The Way To Fitness ÷ presents the latest fitness research available. A first of its kind, this manual will assist individuals like yourself, who are taking physical fitness courses, to understand the basic principles and techniques involved in step training. The added "Plus" in the text tells how to structure a complete physical and mental training workout that will motivate you to make healthy choices for a lifetime.

The book has been developed both for the novice requiring the basics and for the instructor-to-be to understand the methods behind the basics. Its brief, easy-to-follow, sequential learning order can be the map and compass for one's journey toward personal fitness excellence.

Chapter 1 initiates *a step in the right direction* by presenting total fitness principles and definitions. These lay a broad foundation for understanding the specific fitness techniques you will be using. It also will help you describe your starting point — where you are today — through testing procedures that are easily conducted in a class setting. From there, you'll be able to establish program goals, monitor your progress, and see your results.

Chapter 2 encourages you to take the *first step* in understanding the specific fitness activity called step training. It covers the benefits, latest research, how to choose your bench height and music tempo, proper alignment and technique, positions to avoid, and general safety precautions.

Chapter 3 presents the *segments of a step class* and specific information to consider while participating in each. The four segments are: warm-up, step aerobics, strength/isolation training, and the cool-down, flexibility, and relaxation segment.

Chapter 4 takes you *step by step* through the basic techniques of step training. A chapter opening illustration depicts how the steps are classified, clarifying the varieties given. The techniques are described and photographed using the "mirrored" method for all *front* views: A movement described and visualized as using the left foot/arm/or side of the body shown is actually the right foot/arm/side of the model (see Figure I.1). Therefore, you do not have to reverse the direction of what is pictured and what is performed. You simply perform the movement on the same side of the body as you see it photographed and described. (Movement photographed from the model's *side* view or *rear* view are natural and not "mirrored"; right and left steps are the same as model's right and left.)

Creativity is fostered in Chapter 5 by giving you the chance to *step to the beat* — to choreograph your own program. Principles of balance, transitions, and building unlimited possibilities are offered, along with a worksheet to apply what you've learned.

Chapter 6 presents *the next step* — adding variety to your program once you've learned the basics. It first offers ideas on how to safely progress through a step program by varying the intensity so you are suffi-

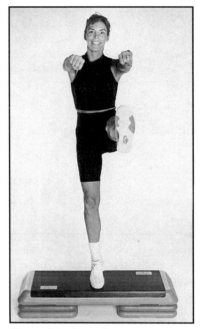

Figure I.1. Stepping up onto the bench, taking weight on your **left** foot, kick your **right** leg forward, waist-high.

ciently and continually challenged according to your own fitness level, skill level, current health status, and goals you've set. Next it covers strength and endurance training of the skeletal muscles using the bench in level, incline, and decline positions, in conjunction with a variety of resistance equipment. Having progressed to being an intermediate-to-advanced stepper, variety in the workout format becomes a plus to stay motivated and to continue adherence to this or any other training modality. The interval step training option combines aerobic stepping and anaerobic strength training in the same routines. We also look briefly at the new two-bench advanced step aerobics challenge and circuit training with bench steps. Each of the three, more advanced options in this chapter can provide a goal for the beginner to aspire to, and that occasional needed change for continually challenging the trained stepper.

Chapter 7 highlights *the balancing step* — healthy choices in other areas of your total fitness program, including establishing the fitness mindset, a program of relaxation, proper nutrition and eating strategies, and weight management techniques.

Chapter 8 sets up the challenge for *future steps*. It presents you with the opportunity to rank your fitness priorities and to establish total program goals toward which to strive.

Enjoy each step of your journey to fitness!

Student Information Profile

Please fill in the following information, remove from the textbook, and give to your instructor:

Name _____Rank: F/So/J/S/Grad/Other

Address _____Phone _____

Social Security No. _____Age_____Height_____Weight_____Ideal Weight_____

Rate Your Fitness Level   **SUPERIOR/EXCELLENT/GOOD**/FAIR/POOR/VERY POOR—PRE

SUPERIOR/EXCELLENT/GOOD/FAIR/POOR/VERY POOR—POST

Previous class or instruction in course: _____

Sports in which you participate/enjoy weekly: _____

Reason(s) for taking course: _____

Did anyone recommend this course or instructor? _____

If so, whom? _____

Physical limitations _____

Activity you would especially like instructor to cover: _____

Heart rate: Resting_____Training Zone _____–_____

List any drug you take (which may alter your heart rate): _____

Do you desire to: (circle) Gain lean weight / Lose fat weight / Stay same

Do you smoke? _____If so, number per day:_____

Rate your alcohol consumption: Never/Daily/Other/ _____

List interests in music, favorite song, favorite artist:_____

Other interests _____

If 35 or older or have specific limitation: I have my doctor's written permission to participate.

Doctor's name and phone: _____

I have read and understand the responsibilities for participants and the instructor.

_____
Signature   Date

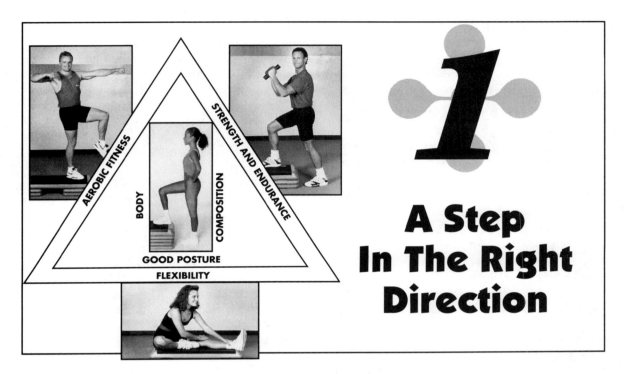

AEROBIC FITNESS

STRENGTH AND ENDURANCE

BODY COMPOSITION

GOOD POSTURE

FLEXIBILITY

A Step In The Right Direction

By engaging in a physical fitness activity such as step training, you've taken the first step toward a meaningful, active lifestyle. Physical conditioning through step aerobics offers you a happier, more vivacious and abundant life. The physically fit active lifestyle actually prolongs life.[1] Furthermore, "Some predictions are that by the end of this century, the average American woman will live to age ninety, and the average American man to the mid-eighties.[2] With these impressive findings and a projected long life ahead of us, let's make sure it will be a *quality* long life we're living (not just doing time), by making good choices.

❖ AEROBIC / STEP AEROBICS

Most simply stated, the term *aerobic* means *promoting the supply and use of oxygen*. The body's demand for oxygen increases when you engage in vigorous activity that produces specific beneficial changes in the body. Aerobic can, therefore, refer to *any type of exercise mode as long as certain basic criteria are met*.

Step training or step *aerobics* is an exercise mode of activity that fulfills all of the criteria for aerobic exercise established by the American College of Sports Medicine.

To clarify, then, *aerobic* is an adjective describing another word, and step *aerobics* is a noun denoting a mode of activity.

❖ A TOTAL PHYSICAL FITNESS CONDITIONING PROGRAM

Total physical fitness is the positive state of well-being allowing you enough strength and energy to participate in a full, active lifestyle of your choice. It is "the general capacity to adapt favorably to physical effort. Individuals are physically fit when they are able to meet both the usual and unusual demands of daily life, safely and effectively without undue stress or exhaustion," according to the American Medical Association.

A total physical fitness conditioning program consists of five basic parts. This can be visualized by the fitness triangle, depicting three action-type components, based on underlying structural components as shown in the chapter opening photos.

1. *Aerobic fitness* (cardiovascular and respiratory)
2. *Flexibility* (ability to bend and stretch)
3. *Muscular strength and muscular endurance* (thickening muscle fiber mass to enable individuals to endure a heavier workload)
4. *Good posture* (holding body in proper position for safety and efficiency)
5. *Body composition* (maintaining proper fat weight-to-lean weight ratio).

1   Aerobic Fitness

A total, well-rounded weekly fitness conditioning program should consist of regular participation in all five components. Because the sign of genuine fitness is the condition of the heart, blood vessels, and lungs, however, aerobic fitness is the most important component. By engaging in step training or any other aerobic activity, the heart gradually strengthens and develops a greater capacity to pump more oxygenated blood to the body with fewer contractions. Exercised hearts are stronger and slower.

> Highly trained and conditioned endurance athletes have resting heart rates as low as 30 to 32 beats per minute, an unbelievably low rate! What actually happens is that with regular, stimulating exercise, the heart becomes a more efficient pump. It pumps more blood with each stroke, and with a more efficient stroke volume, your heart can function with less effort. By getting your heart into condition, you may be practicing preventive medicine. You may be lessening the danger of a coronary heart attack, five, ten, fifteen, twenty years from now. And if you do have one, your chances of surviving are far greater with a heart, lungs, and blood vessels which are in good condition.[3]

A person can exist without big, bulging muscles, or without the perfect figure, or with a head cold, but not very long without a good heart and lungs. Unfortunately, more than 40 percent of all people who have a first heart attack do not have a second chance to change their habits or develop an aerobic program. They die.[4] And more than half of all American deaths each year are attributable to heart-related diseases.[5] If only we could establish a living pattern priority early in life to counteract this overwhelming statistic!

2   Flexibility

Flexibility is defined as *the functional range of motion of a certain joint and its corresponding muscle groups.* The greater the range of movement, the more the muscles, tendons, and ligaments can flex or bend. Muscles are arranged in pairs. One muscle's ability to shorten or contract is directly related to the opposing muscle's length or stretch. Flexibility is maintained or increased by movement patterns that slowly and progressively stretch the muscle beyond its relaxed length. The stretch is performed to a point at which tension developing in the muscle is felt, but not to a point of pain.

3   Muscular Strength and Endurance

Muscular *strength* is the *ability of a muscle to exert a force against a resistance.* Strength activities increase the amount of force muscles can exert, or the amount of work muscles can perform. Activities such as weight training can develop strength in the skeletal muscles.

Muscular *endurance* is the *ability of muscles to work strenuously for relatively long periods without fatigue.* It is the capacity of a muscle to exert a force repeatedly, or to hold a static (still) contraction over time.

Muscular strength and endurance activities do not provide increased oxygen to condition the heart to function more efficiently.[6] Their primary target is skeletal muscle.

4   Good Posture/Good Positioning

Proper positioning of the body when performing any type of physical exertion promotes a safe and efficient workout. Once the basic mechanics are known and practiced, this underlying fitness component becomes an integral part of every move, not a separate program.

5 Body Composition

An individual's total body weight is composed of fat weight and lean weight (fat-free weight). Keeping an appropriate percentage ratio between these two weights is important for the entire body's best functioning and helps prevent obesity and its many related health risks. This fitness component is managed by establishing a proper diet and exercise plan that provides for ideal weight maintenance.

If you aren't beginning your program at an ideal weight, specific guidelines will be given within both the physical exercise programs and the dietary eating plans you'll establish for how to achieve an ideal percentage ratio.

In summation, of the five components involved in developing a total physical fitness conditioning workout program (your *prescription exercise plan*), aerobic fitness training is considered the most important. The remainder of this chapter is devoted to a detailed look at this research and the general principles recommended for you to follow, including modes of activity to choose in addition to step training. The other four physical fitness components are explained more fully in later chapters.

⊹ ▬▬▬▬▬▬▬▬▬▬▬▬▬▬▬
AEROBIC FITNESS TRAINING

AEROBIC CAPACITY IMPROVEMENT: YOUR MAIN OBJECTIVE

Aerobic means promoting the supply and use of oxygen, and training refers to muscle stimulation. Therefore, aerobic training is any exercise that requires a steady supply of oxygen for an extended time and demands an uninterrupted work output from the muscles.

An activity such as step training significantly increases the oxygen supply to all body parts, including the heart and lungs, through continuous, rhythmic movement of large muscles and connective tissue. This type of movement conditions the body's oxygen transport system (heart, lungs, blood, and blood vessels) to process oxygen more efficiently. This *efficiency in processing oxygen*, called *aerobic capacity*, is dependent on your ability to:

⊹ Rapidly breathe large amounts of air.

⊹ Forcefully deliver large volumes of blood.

⊹ Effectively deliver oxygen to all parts of the body.

In short, one's aerobic capacity depends upon efficient lungs, a powerful heart, and a good vascular system. Because it reflects the conditions of these vital organs, *aerobic capacity is the best index (single measure) of overall physical fitness.*[7]

Aerobic capacity is what is measured, quantified, and labeled in a physical fitness stress test, performed either in a laboratory (called a laboratory stress test) or on a pre-measured distance such as a track (called a field stress test). Later in the chapter, you are given the opportunity to test your aerobic capacity using either method.

STRENGTHENING THE HEART: PROGRESSIVE OVERLOAD PRINCIPLE

Step training, or any aerobic activity, conditions the heart muscle by strengthening it through a principle called *progressive overload*. Not only will the heart pump more blood with each beat, but it will also have a longer rest between each beat, thereby lowering the pulse rate. Aerobic exercise overloads the heart by causing it to beat faster during the specific time-frame of the workout session, producing a temporary high demand on the cardiorespiratory system. Over time, as you become more fit, the heart eventually adjusts to this temporary high demand, and soon it is able to do the same amount of work with less effort.

By overloading the heart with any vigorous aerobic exercise, your aerobic capacity increases and a desirable training effect can be achieved. The *training effect*, or total beneficial changes that usually occur, consists of:

⁎ Stronger heart, sending more oxygenated blood to all tissues of the body.

⁎ More blood cells produced.

⁎ Slower resting heart rate.

⁎ Expansion of blood vessels.

⁎ Improvement of muscle tone.

⁎ Lower blood pressure through improved circulation.

⁎ Stronger respiratory muscles.

⁎ Regulation of the release of adrenalin.

⁎ Increased lung capacity.

⁎ More regular elimination of solid wastes.

⁎ Lower levels of fat in blood.[8]

⁎ Strengthening of muscles and skeleton to protect them from injury later in life.

⁎ Deterring osteoporosis by increasing bone density.[9]

⁎ Increased sensitivity to insulin and lowered blood sugar levels in mild, adult-onset diabetes.[10]

⁎ Improvement in the way the body handles cholesterol, by increasing the proportion of blood cholesterol attached to high-density lipoprotein — a carrier molecule that keeps cholesterol from damaging artery walls.[11]

AEROBIC EXERCISE ALTERNATIVES

Aerobic exercise options in addition to bench/step training include all of the following activities:

⁎ Aerobic dance-exercise (aerobics)

⁎ Cross-country skiing

⁎ Cycling (including stationary cycling)

⁎ Jogging/running

⁎ Jumping rope

⁎ Rowing

⁎ Skating (ice/roller/in-line)

⁎ Stair climbing

⁎ Swimming

⁎ Walking/hiking (moderate to fast pace-walk).

AEROBIC CRITERIA

These exercise alternatives, collectively, have several essential criteria for the exercise to be labeled *aerobic* (see Figure 1.1). Because aerobic means *with oxygen*, the movement you do must:

1. *Use the large muscles of the body*,[12] (arms and legs). The gesture and step patterns in bench/step movements are excellent choices.

2. *Be rhythmic*.[13] One-two-one-two, using a steady beat of music, with either a fast or slow tempo, is suggested.

3. *Practice a minimum of three sessions per week*.[14]

⁎ Four days a week or every other day is good.

⁎ Some key researchers recommend five days as a maximum for fitness goals. Beyond this, injuries to the musculoskeletal system from overuse are ten times more likely to occur. Give your body at least two days off per week, especially if you are a novice to physical fitness conditioning.

⁎ If your goals are related to more than just aerobic fitness — if, perhaps, your profession (e.g., fitness instructor) or your athletic sport status requires more workouts or days per week — allow your body to tell you your maximum frequency. A sudden elevated resting heart rate in the morning signifies the day(s) not to work out. This is your built-in body signal, and it can be readily seen/heard/felt simply by daily monitoring your resting heart rate. Upon arising in the morning, check this heart rate for one full minute.

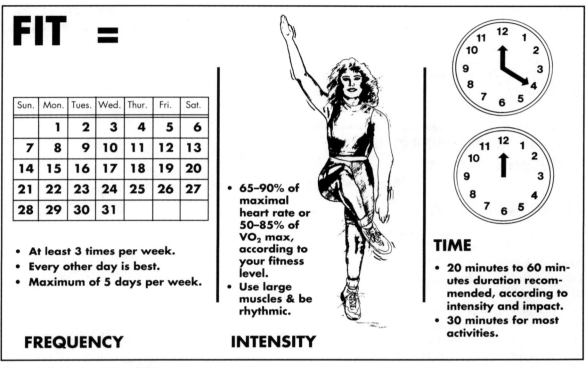

Figure 1.1 Five aerobic criteria.

4. *Exercise continuously for 20-60 minutes.*[15]

   ✛ Duration depends upon the intensity and the impact of the activity. (Both of these terms are explained later in full detail.)

   ✛ Lower intensity activity, such as walking, should be done over a longer period (40-60 minutes).

   ✛ Because high-impact types of activity, such as running and jumping, generally cause significantly more debilitating injuries to exercisers, shorter workouts (20 minutes) are recommended.

5. To receive the cardiorespiratory fitness benefits (called the training effect), *the heart rate must be maintained in a specific target heart rate training zone*, which is the individualized safe pace at which to aerobically work or exercise. This reflects your intensity and is explained scientifically as one of the following:

   ✛ 65-90 percent of your maximum heart rate or

   ✛ 50-85 percent of your maximum oxygen uptake, or heart rate reserve.[16]

INTENSITY DETAILED

Frequency and time duration of your workouts are easy to determine but the amount of exertion during the workout to keep it safe while continually making fitness gains can be more of a challenge to determine, especially for the novice. Intensity is measured (monitored) in one of three ways:

✛ Finding your target heart rate (THR) training zone using the Karvonen formula. This is suggested for the novice.

✛ Using the psychophysical scale for ratings of perceived exertion (RPE), which shows a high correlation with heart rate and other metabolic parameters, according to American College of Sports Medicine (ACSM) guidelines. Rate of perceived exertion monitoring is suggested for the individual who already has become well-accustomed to taking a heart rate pulse.

❖ Using the talk test. This easy and practical method is best used in conjunction with the THR and RPE for monitoring exercise intensity.

❖ YOUR TARGET HEART RATE TRAINING ZONE

TAKING YOUR PULSE

To calculate appropriate exercise intensity using this method, you first must know how to accurately take your pulse. The pulse equals heartbeats per minute and can be felt and counted at one of six pulsation points. Select which area you can best obtain a pulse using your index and second fingers. The two places most often used to count pulse are the neck near the carotid artery and the wrist near the radial artery. Both are shown in Figure 1.2.

1. The carotid artery, located in the neck, is usually easy to find. Place your index and middle fingers below the point of your jawbone and slide downward an inch or so, pressing lightly. When you use the carotid artery pulse-monitoring method, make sure to apply light pressure, as excessive pressure may cause the heart rate to slow down by a reflex action.

2. The radial artery extends up the wrist on the thumb side. Place your index and middle fingers just below the base of your thumb. Press lightly. Count the number of pulsations, or beats, for 60 seconds. The total is the number of heartbeats per minute. To count correctly, make sure you count each beat you feel.

Having gained the skill of pulse taking, it is now time to establish your *resting heart rate*. This number is to be placed in the formula for establishing your target heart rate training zone.

Monitoring the Resting Heart Rate

A true *resting* heart rate (RsHR) is not taken in a class but, instead, when the individual has been at complete rest, preferably after sleeping for several hours and upon awakening. Keep a clock or watch with a second hand next to your bed. When you awaken (without an alarm clock ring), take your pulse for one full minute and record that number as your RsHR. Do this for five consecutive mornings, then determine an average (add all RsHR's and divide by 5). This is a rather accurate determination of your resting heart rate.

NOTE: Unusual stress and illness (illness is a type of stress) sharply elevate the resting heart rate from previous readings.

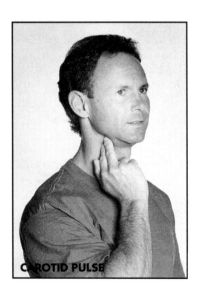
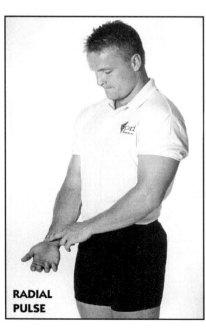

CAROTID PULSE

RADIAL PULSE

Figure 1.2. Taking the carotid pulse and the radial pulse.

Normally healthy individuals should find a positive outlet for stress. Stress affects you even as you sleep (constant rapid heart rate), a time when the heart ideally should take a break and slow down for six to eight hours.

One of the two visible signs of improvement in heart and lung fitness is a lower resting heart rate. Because the RsHR is the basic thermometer of fitness, after a ten-to-fifteen-week step aerobics course, you and your classmates may experience:

✧ An average –3 heartbeats per minute resting heart rate decline.

✧ An average –10 heartbeats per minute by smokers who quit (or significantly change their consumption) during the course and as much as a –24 heartbeats per minute decline.[17]

Determining Your Target Heart Rate Training Zone

Your average RsHR figure is now placed in the formula for determining your target heart rate training zone. See Table 1.1, Section 3. The other variables figured into the formula are current age and lifestyle, represented as a percentage of maximum heart rate.

If you are:	Use:
✧ a non-athletic adult	50% to begin
✧ sedentary	60-69%
✧ moderately active	70-75%
✧ very active and well-trained	80-85%

Record your age and the selected percentage range from above that describes your lifestyle. Figure the Karvonen equation. The result is your target heart rate, the safe exercise training zone for you.

Taking a Count After a Step Aerobics Interval

As you are beginning a step aerobics program, you will want to monitor your pace several times during the workout hour so you can learn constant endurance pacing. Mentally remember your readings, and record them at the end of class.

When you take a pulse rate during the learning process and find that your pace is below your established training zone, increase your intensity. If you have a pulse rate higher than your established training zone, lower your intensity.

To become familiar with your own response to various intensity levels so you can better regulate yourself, ask yourself, "How do I feel when I get this pulse?" Focus not only on your pulse count but also on what feelings and conditions the number relates to, so you can begin to recognize the signals your body sends. This also will help prepare you to use the RPE monitoring method of intensity, which, as you become a more advanced exerciser, will be a more practical and practiced method than counting your heartbeats per minute.

Continuing at a pace that is too intense will prove to be an anaerobic exercise program. Anaerobic activity is basically stop and start, in which the heart is not kept at a constant, steady pace for 20 to 60 minutes. Thus, anaerobic describes an activity that requires all-out effort of short duration and does not utilize oxygen to produce energy. This type of exercise quickly uses up more oxygen than the body can take in while engaging in the exercise, causing an oxygen debt. This, in turn, causes lactic acids (waste products) to accumulate in the muscles, which leads to exhaustion.

The pulse-monitoring procedure during step aerobics is then to slow down, walk around, find your pulse, and count it for either 6 or 10 seconds. Each of these counts has been found to be a scientifically accurate measurement for aerobic activity pulse rates. Taking a timed count of greater than 10 seconds immediately after aerobic exercise will tend to be inaccurate because the heart rate slows down to a recovery pulse rather rapidly. You or your instructor will determine whether you will count for 6 or 10 seconds. Immediately following the aerobic exercise segment, count your pulse and multiply the number you get times 10 if using the 6-second count, or times 6 if using a 10-second count. Each of these newly multiplied numbers

TABLE 1.1

How to Figure Your Target Heart Rate Training Zone

As three basic factors enter into figuring your estimated safe exercise zone, those must be established first:

1. Your current age: _____

2. How active is your lifestyle? _____% MHR. If you are:

    (Choose one:)

    ÷ Non-athletic adult: use 50% of your maximum heart rate.
    ÷ Sedentary: use the figure 60–69% of your maximum heart rate (but only for the first two or three weeks).
    ÷ Moderately physically active: use 70–75% of your maximum heart rate.
    ÷ Active and well-trained: use 80–85% of your maximum heart rate.

3. Your average resting heart rate:_____

Now place your numbers in the Karvonen formula, which follows:

A. 220   – _____ = _____**Estimated Maximal Heart Rate (MHR)**
    (Index number)   **(Your Age)**

B. _____ – _____ = _____
       MHR   **Resting HR**   **HR Reserve**

C._____ × . _____ = _____ + **Resting HR** = _____*
  Heart Rate Reserve   **Lower end lifestyle activity range**
               (i.e., #2 above)

  _____ × . _____ = _____ + **Resting HR** = _____*
  Heart Rate Reserve   **Higher end lifestyle activity range**
               (i.e., #2 above)

RANGE (vertical, right side)

RANGE OF   _____*   This range is your estimated safe exercise zone. Keep your heart rate
YOUR   working in this range while you aerobically exercise for approximately
TARGET   _____* 30 minutes of each session.

                                 Re-figure as you "age," as you can reclassify your "lifestyle" of activity,
                                 or as your resting heart rate markedly declines.

For example: Chris is 20 years old, a moderately active person (70–75% range), with a resting heart rate of 62.

A. 220 − 20 = 200 MHR

B. 200 − 62 = 138 Heart Rate Reserve

C. 138 × .70 = 96 + 62 = 158*
   138 × .75 = 104 + 62 = 166*   ) Target Heart Rate Training Zone

If Chris keeps working (aerobically exercising) at the range of 158 to 166 heartbeats per minute, the heart will be safely working toward the training effect.

will equal heartbeats per minute and hopefully will always be in your training zone.

NOTE: Taking a 6-second count is easy. All you do is add a zero to the pulse you feel, and record that number. You must carefully begin and end exactly with a timer.

Table 1.2 lists target heart rate counts for individuals who wish to attain fitness using the ideal aerobic range for most people (60-75% of heart rate reserve). Locate the column across the top that is closest to your age and the row down the left side reflecting a figure closest to your resting heart rate. The box where the column and row intersect is *your 10-second target heart rate training zone.*

As your cardiorespiratory system becomes more fit and efficient, work (exercise) will become easier, and you will have to increase the intensity of your activities. Techniques for increasing and decreasing the intensity of your workout will be explained later. By using the target heart rate training zone, you automatically compensate for increased fitness and still maintain the same training effect. Thus, your heart rate will increase during the vigorous aerobic step training activity and should return to normal (pre-activity heart rate) within a short time after the workout. As a rule, the faster it slows down (recovers from exercise), the more physically fit you are, for recovery heart rate improvement is another indication of increased fitness level.

TABLE 1.2   Target Heart Rate Training Zones*

Your Age ▶

Your Av. Resting Heart Rate ▼	15	20	25	30	35	40	45	50	55	60	65	70	75	80
90	27-29	26-29	26-28	25-28	25-27	24-26	23-26	23-25	22-24	22-24	21-23	21-22	20-22	20-21
85	26-29	26-29	25-28	25-27	24-27	24-26	23-25	23-25	22-24	22-24	21-23	21-22	20-22	20-21
80	26-29	25-28	25-28	24-27	24-26	23-26	23-25	22-25	22-24	21-23	21-23	20-22	20-21	19-21
75	26-29	25-28	25-28	24-27	24-26	23-26	23-25	22-25	21-24	21-23	20-23	20-22	19-21	19-21
70	25-29	25-28	24-27	24-27	23-26	23-25	22-25	22-24	21-24	21-24	20-22	20-22	19-21	19-20
65	25-28	25-28	24-27	23-26	23-26	22-25	21-24	21-24	21-23	20-23	20-22	19-21	19-21	18-20
60	25-28	24-28	24-27	23-26	23-26	22-25	21-24	21-24	20-23	20-22	19-22	19-21	18-21	18-20
55	24-27	23-27	23-27	23-26	22-25	21-24	21-24	21-24	20-23	20-22	19-22	19-21	18-20	18-20
50	24-28	23-27	23-26	22-26	22-25	21-25	21-24	20-23	20-23	19-22	19-21	18-21	18-20	17-20

*The numbers in the squares represent pulse beats counted in ten seconds.

THE BORG SCALE: RATINGS OF PERCEIVED EXERTION

The second method for monitoring intensity utilizes the psychophysical Borg scale for ratings of perceived exertion (RPE),[18] as shown in Table 1.3.

This scale is based on the finding that, while exercising, one has the ability to accurately assess how hard the body is working. It is basically a judgment call and is more appropriate when used by individuals who have been exercising for a while. The untrained exerciser typically reports a higher RPE than an athlete, at the same exercise heart rate.

RPE seems to correlate strongly with other workload indicators, such as ventilation, oxygen consumption, and muscle metabolism. Participants tune into the overall sensation of effort exerted by their entire body, rather than one factor such as local calf or hamstring exhaustion, panting, sweating, or body temperature. When used along with heart rate monitoring, RPE is useful for the novice, who may not yet be aware of how exercise is supposed to feel.

You might begin to make mental notes to yourself during the workout hour concerning your ratings of perceived exertion. After the workout, immediately record what you felt for each phase of the workout, expressed as numbers from 0 to 10.

TABLE 1.3. Borg Scale Ratings of Perceived Exertion[18]

Rating	WHAT IS FELT	PHASE OF PROGRAM
0.5	"Very, Very Light; Just Noticeable"	
1	"Very Light"	Warm-Up Phase
2	"Light (Weak)"	marginally conducive to the development of cardio-respiratory endurance.
3	"Moderate"	When you exercise below this level, the exercise stimulus is only... / For aerobic fitness, if you can sing here, you need to work harder. (Cool-Down Phase)
4	"Somewhat Hard"	3–5 ACSM Recommended "Aerobics" Range[2] — Feel as if you could maintain the intensity for a long time while thinking, talking with a partner, or enjoying the class or scenery.
5	"Heavy / Strong"	"Peak aerobic dance-exercise"
6		
7	"Very Hard"	Pulse races and it become difficult to say more than a few words for prolonged periods of time. There is a sense that this level of intensity cannot last.
8		
9		
10	"Very, Very Hard; Almost Maximum; Exhaustion."	The end of a competitive race or sprint interval.

Begin to notice the correlation between target heart rates achieved and how ratings of perceived exertion feel.

THE TALK TEST

A third and less formal method for determining aerobic intensity is called the *talk test*. It is based on the premise that, while exercising, the participant should always be able to hold a conversation. If the participant can gasp out only one or two words at a time, the exercise intensity is probably anaerobic and should be adjusted to allow for two- to three-word phrases. Because the accuracy of the talk test varies within any given population, it is best utilized in conjunction with the THR and the RPE for monitoring exercise intensity.[19]

WHICH METHOD IS BEST?

The experts do not agree when it comes to THR versus RPE. Some claim that only THR methods are accurate; others believe that RPE and the talk test are more practical. Because all the methods are useful and none is consistently ideal, a good solution is to *use a combination of all three*. Once a participant has developed a good understanding of the heart rate/RPE relationship, heart rate can be monitored less frequently and RPE can be used as a primary means of measuring exercise intensity with the talk test as an informal supplemental backup measure.[20]

✤ ▬▬▬▬▬▬▬▬▬▬
FITNESS TESTING DETERMINES YOUR STARTING POINT

The next step in the journey toward achieving and then maintaining physical fitness for a lifetime involves establishing your current fitness starting point, using scientific test and assessment procedures. Clearly knowing yourself in terms of your past history, risk factors, and present physical status will assist you in developing a lifetime

fitness plan. It will enable you to not only realistically and safely set achievable short-term fitness goals but also will provide the basis for continually motivating you to adhere to the program you do establish to achieve your long-range and lifetime fitness goals.

You initially may find that it can be painful and devastating to realize you are out of shape and test poorly on a laboratory or field stress test. No one really wants to see scientific results that label him or her inferior or below the norm. But having the determination and courage to find out just where you are at the outset and then, with time and dedication, progressing to the point where your post-assessment test numbers represent an excellent state of fitness and well-being, is motivating!

In most instances, specific fitness testing is appropriate only after obtaining a medical history. Screening may uncover any potential problems and determine if you should be considered for a specific exercise prescription. Most course settings require this pre-screening, or a thorough medical exam if you have any limitations or known risk factors.

UNDERSTANDING FITNESS ASSESSMENTS

The purpose of an initial pre-course fitness assessment is to *establish a baseline of information from which later changes can be compared*. Assessment principles include the following:

1. Testing is an effective way to measure your improvement in performance over time and not as an absolutely correct physiologic measurement or comparison.

2. By following consistent procedures of testing (using the same test, person administering it, instrument, time of day, etc.), you are more assured of accuracy in measurement over time.

3. Results are recorded for comparison purposes. The person being tested should understand these values and ask questions as needed to ensure understanding.

MEASURING AEROBIC CAPACITY

Pre-assessing your current status by having a thorough physical fitness exam will measure your heart's response to increasing amounts of exercise (work, stress) by measuring your ability to use oxygen. Physical fitness can and should be measured in one of two ways at least every three years:

❖ A laboratory physical fitness test.

❖ A field test administered by you and a friend.

THE LABORATORY PHYSICAL FITNESS TEST

The "master key" to good health and exercising without fear is a properly conducted treadmill stress test to check out the precise condition of your heart.[21] Physical fitness and health are different, and the treadmill stress ECG helps to make that distinction.[22]

Prior to a treadmill stress test, you will be thoroughly screened. This consists of: (a) a brief history-taking and physical exam during which the technician listens to your heart and lungs; (b) a check for the use of drugs known to affect the ECG (e.g., various heart and hypertensive medications); (c) a check for history of congenital or acquired heart disorders; and (d) an evaluation of the resting ECG.

This screening and background check will help to determine your risk factors. A risk factor is a feature in a person's heredity, background, or present lifestyle that increases the likelihood of developing coronary heart disease. If no risk factors are present, an exercise test usually is not necessary below age thirty-five if guidelines mentioned earlier are followed. If symptoms of heart, lung, or metabolic disease are present, a maximum stress test is recommended for individuals of any age prior to the onset of a vigorous exercise program, and followed with tests every two years.[23]

Sub-Maximal Testing

Sub-maximal testing is accomplished by means of a physical fitness test (stress test) on a treadmill. Electrocardiogram leads transmit and record electrical (heart) impulses that are read on a machine and recorded on a strip of paper. You are tested only to approximately 150 beats per minute, not to exhaustion.

The ECG electrodes with leads are circular rubber discs with wires attached to them. The discs are glued onto the chest and back at key locations so various "pictures" of your heart, from different angles and sides, can all be recorded at once. Usually between seven and ten electrodes are applied, depending on the laboratory's procedures or on the individual's specific needs.

You probably will be asked to walk at a pace of 3.3 miles per hour (90 meters per minute) on the treadmill. The grade will begin flat and will increase slowly in gradation, as if you were walking up a hill. Every minute the "hill" will become steeper and more difficult to climb. When your heart rate reaches 150 beats per minute, a record is made of the amount of time it took for you to arrive at that reading. Then, through an indirect method of extrapolation (projection of maximum results from having tested many others the same way in the past), your fitness ability is estimated.

Basically, the longer your heart rate takes to reach 150 beats per minute, the more fit you are; the shorter, the less fit you are. Sub-maximal fitness testing usually is used with those who know of no outstanding limitations and who are interested in starting an aerobic step training program.

Maximal Testing

Maximal testing procedures are administered if an individual's need is more specific (i.e., for diagnostic or research purposes). Maximum testing directly reveals how much oxygen you use, because you are tested to exhaustion. The "exhaustion" point is when you start to get markedly fatigued. Some researchers believe that maximum laboratory testing is the *only* conclusive type to use.

FIELD TESTS OF FITNESS

You may not have immediate access to a laboratory and qualified physiologists to monitor the results recorded with the treadmill method. Therefore, field tests have been developed to help you assess your own physical fitness by determining your current aerobic capacity. This testing is easily conducted in an aerobics class setting.

The following information and Tables 1.4 and 1.5 were developed from Dr. Kenneth Cooper's book, *The Aerobics Program for Total Well-Being.*[24] Cooper's 12-Minute Test and 1.5-Mile Test are two that you can administer by yourself or with the help of a friend. You should assess your cardiorespiratory endurance using one of these tests before you begin your step aerobics program, and reassess your cardiorespiratory efficiency eight weeks later. As step aerobics becomes a lifetime activity for you, an ongoing assessment should be done every two months, and your results compared with those from your first assessment. This also will help you set continual, lifelong, specific physical fitness goals.

TABLE 1.4   Cooper's 12-Minute Walking/Running Test: Distance (Miles) Covered in 12 Minutes

Fitness Category		Age (years)					
		13-19	20-29	30-39	40-49	50-59	60 +
I. Very Poor	(men)	<1.30	<1.22	<1.18	<1.14	<1.03	< .87
	(women)	< 1.0	< .96	< .94	< .88	< .84	< .78
II. Poor	(men)	1.30-1.37	1.22-1.31	1.18-1.30	1.14-1.24	1.03-1.16	.87-1.02
	(women)	1.00-1.18	.96-1.11	.95-1.05	.88- .98	.84- .93	.78- .86
III. Fair	(men)	1.38-1.56	1.32-1.49	1.31-1.45	1.25-1.39	1.17-1.30	1.03-1.20
	(women)	1.19-1.29	1.12-1.22	1.06-1.18	.99-1.11	.94-1.05	.87- .98
IV. Good	(men)	1.57-1.72	1.50-1.64	1.46-1.56	1.40-1.53	1.31-1.44	1.21-1.32
	(women)	1.30-1.43	1.23-1.34	1.19-1.29	1.12-1.24	1.06-1.18	.99-1.09
V. Excellent	(men)	1.73-1.86	1.65-1.76	1.57-1.69	1.54-1.65	1.45-1.58	1.33-1.55
	(women)	1.44-1.51	1.35-1.45	1.30-1.39	1.25-1.34	1.19-1.30	1.10-1.18
VI. Superior	(men)	>1.87	>1.77	>1.70	>1.66	>1.59	>1.56
	(women)	>1.52	>1.46	>1.40	>1.35	>1.31	>1.19

< Means less than; > more than.

From *The Aerobics Program For Total Well-Being,* by Kenneth H. Cooper, M.D., M.P.H., Copyright 1982 by Kenneth H. Cooper. Reprinted by permission of the publisher, Bantam-Doubleday-Dell, New York, NY 10103.

Cooper's 12-Minute Test Results

PRE-TEST:

Start Time: _____ Stop Time: _____ Distance Covered: _____

Check Table 1.4 for Fitness Category.

Circle Fitness Category: Very Poor / Poor / Fair / Good / Excellent / Superior   **GOAL:** _____

POST-TEST:

Start Time: _____ Stop Time: _____ Distance Covered: _____

Check Table 1.4 for Fitness Category.

Circle Fitness Category: Very Poor / Poor / Fair / Good / Excellent / Superior   **GOAL:** _____

NOTE: If you are over age thirty-five, you should start a step aerobics program by first seeing your doctor and then taking a monitored laboratory fitness test. Individuals with known cardiovascular, pulmonary, or metabolic disease should have a maximum stress test prior to beginning vigorous exercise at any age. These people and those whose exercise tests are abnormal should get a stress test annually.

As guidelines for field testing:

1. If you previously have been physically inactive, participate in one to two weeks of walking or beginning step aerobics before undertaking either of Cooper's tests.

2. Wear loose clothing in which you can freely sweat, and a sport shoe (such as a "cross-trainer").

3. Determine first which field test you plan to take. You can choose running with time or distance as the stopping point.
   - ⁝⁚ If time is the stopping point, take the 12-minute test.
   - ⁝⁚ If distance is the stopping point, take the 1.5-mile test.
   - ⁝⁚ If you believe rather strongly that you are really out of shape, the 12-minute test will be easier because you run for this amount of time only. (An individual might take 20 minutes to complete 1.5 miles.)

4. Be sure you have a stopwatch or a second-hand on your watch, or that you are close to a wall timer.

5. Immediately before performing the test, spend 5 to 10 minutes warming up the muscles (see Chapter 3).

6. Have a partner record your data (as time it takes or laps or distance).

7. Run or walk (or a combination) as quickly as you can for 12 minutes or 1.5 miles. (See Figure 1.3). This is an all-out test of endurance.

8. When you stop, identify precisely the distance covered in miles and tenths of miles or time it took, and have your partner record it.

9. Be sure to cool down by first walking slowly for several minutes, and then finish by doing cool-down stretching.

10. Interpret your results for the specific test you used, on Tables 1.4 or 1.5. At the conclusion of your course, reassess your fitness. What change did you experience from the Pre-Test to Post-Test?

For some beginners, the "good" performance level is high. Do not be discouraged. You will be pleased with your improvement as you participate in a regular step aerobics program.

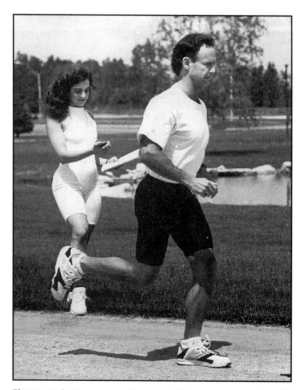

Figure 1.3 Run or walk as quickly as you can for 12 minutes or 1.5 miles.

TABLE 1.5 Cooper's 1.5-Mile Run/Walk Test Time (Minutes)[24]

Fitness Category		Age (years)					
		13-19	20-29	30-39	40-49	50-59	60 +
I. Very Poor	(men)	>15:31	>16:01	>16:31	>17:31	>19:01	>20:01
	(women)	>18:31	>19:01	>19:31	>20:01	>20:31	>21:01
II. Poor	(men)	12:11-15:30	14:01-16:00	14:44-16:30	15:36-17:30	17:01-19:00	19:01-20:00
	(women)	16:55-18:30	18:31-19:00	19:01-19:30	19:31-20:00	20:01-20:30	21:00-21:31
III. Fair	(men)	10:49-12:10	12:01-14:00	12:31-14:45	13:01-15:35	14:31-17:00	16:16-19:00
	(women)	14:31-16:54	15:55-18:30	16:31-19:00	17:31-19:30	19:01-20:00	19:31-20:30
IV. Good	(men)	9:41-10:48	10:46-12:00	11:01-12:30	11:31-13:00	12:31-14:30	14:00-16:15
	(women)	12:30-14:30	13:31-15:54	14:31-16:30	15:56-17:30	16:31-19:00	17:31-19:30
V. Excellent	(men)	8:37- 9:40	9:45-10:45	10:00-11:00	10:30-11:30	11:00-12:30	11:15-13:59
	(women)	11:50-12:29	12:30-13:30	13:00-14:30	13:45-15:55	14:30-16:30	16:30-17:30
VI. Superior	(men)	< 8:37	< 9:45	<10:00	<10:30	<11:00	<11:15
	(women)	<11:50	<12:30	<13:00	<13:45	<14:30	<16:30

< Means less than; > more than.

From *The Aerobics Program For Total Well-Being*, by Kenneth H. Cooper, M.D., M.P.H., Copyright 1982 by Kenneth H. Cooper. Reprinted by permission of the publisher, Bantam-Doubleday-Dell, New York, NY 10103.

Cooper's 1.5-Mile Test Results

PRE-TEST:

Check Off Laps: (i.e., 14 for 190-yd. track; 21 for 126-yd. track):

1 - 2 - 3 - 4 - 5 - 6 - 7 - 8 - 9 - 10 - 11 - 12 - 13 - 14 - 15 - 16 - 17 - 18 - 19 - 20 - 21

Time: _____ OR: Just record here if using an open roadway.

Stop Time: _____

–Start Time: _____

Time: _____

Check Table 1.5 for Fitness Category.

Circle Fitness Category: Very Poor / Poor / Fair / Good / Excellent / Superior **GOAL:** _____

POST-TEST:

Check Off Laps: (i.e., 14 for 190-yd. track; 21 for 126-yd. track):

1 - 2 - 3 - 4 - 5 - 6 - 7 - 8 - 9 - 10 - 11 - 12 - 13 - 14 - 15 - 16 - 17 - 18 - 19 - 20 - 21

Time: _____ OR: Just record here if using an open roadway.

Stop Time: _____

–Start Time: _____

Time: _____

Check Table 1.5 for Fitness Category.

Circle Fitness Category: Very Poor / Poor / Fair / Good / Excellent / Superior **GOAL:** _____

FITNESS FOR LIFE

Attaining a level of physical fitness labeled "good" or "high" (lab tests), or "good," "excellent," or "superior" (field tests) does not mean you have achieved a finished product or goal. Instead, you have found a method of getting in shape that must be continued for the rest of your life. If you discontinue your program completely, all your aerobic gains will be lost in 10 weeks.[25]

The need for personal fitness must result in a complete change in lifestyle. You must prioritize and program exercise into your busy weekly schedule for the rest of your life. A "yo-yo" concept of a 10-week class now, and maybe one a year later, just doesn't maintain fitness and a healthy heart.

TOTAL PHYSICAL FITNESS: A CHOICE

You have just completed assessing your aerobic capacity. With this information, you can establish your cardiovascular fitness goals. Setting goals helps to keep you focused on daily improvement and positive change. It encourages consistency in your fitness program and helps to keep you on target because without goals there's nothing to shoot for.

Write one fitness goal to be achieved by the end of this course. Truly stretch yourself and your potential in regard to what you actually are capable of achieving.

Achieving physical fitness requires dedication to personal excellence. There are few shortcuts but many pleasurable alternatives. Once achieved, you must continue to make choices that maintain your fitness for a lifetime. Fitness is a journey — a continual process — not just one destination. Maintaining fitness is a lot easier than initially achieving it, though you also will discover that the less physically fit you are, the longer you will take to become fit.

The total physical fitness journey requires:

❖ seeking valid information;

❖ establishing your starting points;

❖ setting reasonable and challenging goals;

❖ monitoring your daily progress;

❖ continually making self-disciplined choices.

Enjoy the journey!

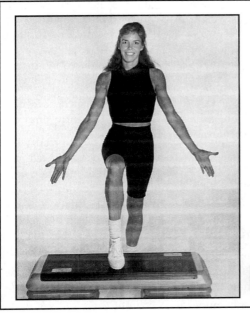

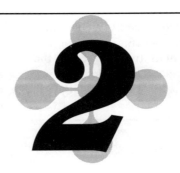

The First Step: Becoming The Informed Stepper

The first step in your journey to fitness is finding and becoming efficient at an exercise activity that is fun, safe, and provides many challenges — generally one that meets all your fitness needs. Bench/step training can be that choice. Because it is a relatively unexplored new training modality with little research so far, all of the related problems and injuries have not yet been fully assessed. To date, the following information and guidelines have been presented by various researchers promoting the activity and companies promoting products to use with the activity.[1, 2, 3, 4, 5]

❖ STEP BENEFITS

Step training involves stepping up and down on a platform or bench, adding a variety of upper torso movements for further challenge. It is known by many names, including bench or step aerobics, bench or step training, bench stepping, and stepping.

The key advantage to a step training program over other aerobics is that it is primarily a high-intensity activity used to promote cardiorespiratory fitness but with low impact for safety

concerns, as a vast majority of all the moves can involve one foot supporting your weight, either on the bench platform or on the floor. Other benefits include the following:

❖ It's a terrific conditioning workout for every major muscle group in the lower body, specifically the hamstrings, quadriceps, gluteals, and calves.

❖ Upper torso movements may provide conditioning work for muscles of the arms, shoulders, chest, and back, and therefore a balanced and complete workout that strengthens and tones the entire body. This becomes especially apparent later if you advance to using 1–4 pound light hand weights in conjunction with your stepping moves.

❖ This workout is unique in its aerobics class versatility. The basic moves are simple, and by introducing various step patterns with fewer (or more) arm gestures, adjusting the height of the bench, or adding or omitting hand weights, participants of all ages, skill and fitness levels, and both genders can be challenged simultaneously.

⋅⋅⋅ **As an effective cardiovascular workout, it has aerobic benefits equal to running 7 miles per hour (mph), yet has the potentially low-impact equivalence of walking at a 3 mph pace, minimizing the chance of injury.**[6]

RESEARCH FINDINGS

Step training is similar to all other forms of physical activity because it has an element of risk. The concerns and subsequent research associated with this new modality of exercise have focused on evaluating:

1. energy cost of aerobic bench/step techniques;

2. physiological benefits;

3. musculoskeletal safety of step training exercise.[7, 8, 9, 10, 11, 12]

The results of research to date include the following highlights:

⋅⋅⋅ Step training provides the sufficient cardiovascular demands needed to attain cardiorespiratory fitness in accordance with American College of Sports Medicine (ACSM) guidelines.

⋅⋅⋅ Determining exact energy costs depends upon various factors including height of the step bench, rate of stepping, and step pattern/technique.

⋅⋅⋅ Bench step height and rate of stepping significantly affect metabolic cost. This varies among participants because of differences in muscle mass rather than height of participants.[13]

⋅⋅⋅ Specific step moves used within a workout all have specific effects on energy cost (i.e., different movement patterns result in different intensities perceived or achieved). For example, moves such as the basic step, step touch, and bypass moves expend less energy than lunging, traveling, and repeater moves.[14]

⋅⋅⋅ Risk of injury involved in this new fitness activity also has been a critical concern. Because research on injuries is gathered over

time, conclusive data are not yet available. Theoretically, it has the potential for injury, but to date no evidence has been found for injury risk any higher than that reported for dance-exercise in general.

In summary, and in keeping with current research data, step training performed according to ACSM guidelines can significantly improve one's cardiovascular fitness. And because several variables can affect heart rate intensity, programs can be designed to continually meet the needs of each individual participant, to facilitate both optimum safety and effectiveness.

CHOOSING YOUR BENCH HEIGHT

When choosing a bench height, consider each of the following factors by referring to the chapter opening photo:

⋅⋅⋅ As a beginner who has not exercised regularly, has limited coordination, or has no experience in step training, you should select a 4" to 6" bench initially. (For the 12" bench shown, this represents the basic 4" platform, and at most, one 2" support block on each end.)

⋅⋅⋅ As an intermediate, or regular step trainer with a "physically fit" level of cardiorespiratory fitness, choose an 8" to 10" bench. (An 8" bench equals the platform plus two 2" support blocks; or, for a 10" bench, three 2" support blocks).

⋅⋅⋅ As an advanced, or skilled regular step trainer with a high level of cardiovascular fitness, choose a 10" to 12" bench (the platform plus a maximum of four support blocks on each end).

⋅⋅⋅ If you are taller or have longer legs than most people, consider using a bench of 8" to 12".

⋅⋅⋅ Regardless of level of fitness or experience, do not select a bench height that allows the knee to flex less than 90 degrees (Figure 2.1) when the knee is weight-bearing. If the knees advance *beyond your toes* as you step up, the platform is too high.

Choosing a platform that is too high for your energy or fitness level may affect your body

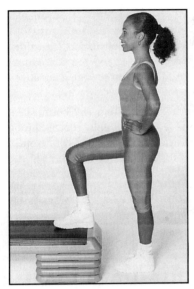

Figure 2.1. If the knees advance beyond your toes as you step up, the platform is too high.

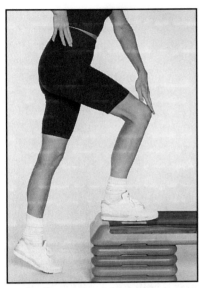

Figure 2.2. Allow a 3" drop from the hip to knee.

alignment and result in injury. For example, if you are leaning too far forward, the platform may be too high and can cause undesirable pressure on the lower back.[15] An optional test for bench height is shown in Figure 2.2: Place one foot flat on top of the bench; allow a 3" drop from the hip to knee for safe movement up to the top of the bench.

MUSIC

Music plays a significant role, as the underlying structure of a step training program. Fun and exciting music can motivate and challenge participants. The tempo of the music (measured as beats per minute) directs the progression of movement and also the speed of the movements. Movements have to be controlled, and music with a BPM (beats per minute) of 118 to 125 is best.[16] For a more advanced workout, **depending on the movements**, 135 bpm may be possible, but proper body alignment and stepping technique are extremely important.[17]

The music should have a clear beat that is easy to follow. Following are the suggested tempos and segment durations.[18]

Duration/mins.	Segment	BPM
10 minutes	Warm-Up	130–140
20–40 minutes	Aerobic Stepping	118–128
3–5 minutes	Aerobic Cool-Down	118–120
10–15 minutes	Isolation	120–130
5–10 minutes	Slow Stretch	<100

BODY ALIGNMENT AND STEPPING TECHNIQUE

Good posture is required for a safe, injury-free workout. Proper alignment and stepping technique include the following:

❖ Keep your back straight, head and chest up, shoulders back, abdomen tight, and buttocks tucked under hips, with eyes on the platform (Figure 2.3).

❖ As much as possible, keep your shoulders aligned over your hips. Lean forward with the whole body. Don't bend from the hips or round the shoulders and lean forward or backward.

❖ Step up lightly, making sure the whole foot lands on the platform, with the heel bearing your weight. Partial foot placement on the bench (with the heel off the bench) increases your chance of slipping off the bench, tripping, or even flipping the bench.

❖ Keep your knees aligned over your feet when they're pulling your body weight onto the platform.

❖ At the top, straighten your legs but don't lock your knees. Keep them "soft."

❖ As you step down, stay close to the platform. Step down, not back. Land on the ball of the foot (Figure 2.4), then bring the heel down onto the floor before taking the next step. Stepping too far back with the leading leg causes the body to lean slightly forward, placing extra stress on the foot, achilles, and calf.

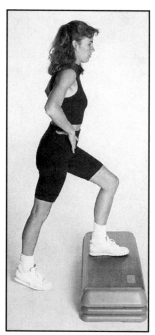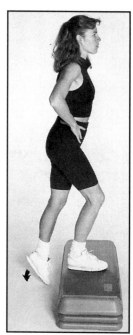

Figure 2.3.　　　　　　**Figure 2.4**
Proper technique for stepping up and stepping down.

Step Carefully

❖ Avoid excessive arm movements over your head.

❖ Maintain appropriate speed for safe and effective movement.

❖ Do not perform more than 8 counts (4 repeaters) on one leg at a time, as repeated foot impact without variation is potentially harmful.

❖ Do not pivot or twist the knee on the weight-bearing leg.

❖ Do not step up with your back toward the platform.

❖ Limit propulsions and power moves.

❖ Maintain muscular balance, working opposing muscle groups equally (quadriceps/hamstrings; calves/tibialis anterior; pectorals/upper back).

❖ If you are pregnant, check with your doctor before starting this program. If you are cleared by your doctor, make certain that you keep your heart rate at 23 beats or below for a 10-second count. A step height of no more than 6" is recommended during pregnancy.

❖ If you feel faint or dizzy or if any exercise causes pain or severe discomfort, stop the exercise immediately but continue to move around.

❖ Do not allow anyone to perform on the bench with you. Only one person at a time should use the bench.

❖ For the bench shown in the chapter opening photo, do not use more than four support blocks on each end of the platform.

Lifting and Lowering

❖ *Do* use correct bench lifting and lowering techniques.

To protect your muscles and joints (especially the lower back) from undue strain or fatigue, proper, efficient technique in these areas must become second nature to you. Disciplined practice of correct techniques now will establish good habits for the rest of your life. The leg muscles are

❖ CORRECT STEP TRAINING POSTURE

Figures 2.5–2.10

Here are three common step training errors to avoid. The man is demonstrating incorrect postural techniques for each exercise, and the woman is performing correctly. Additional performance suggestions are also given.[19]

These moves are important to include for muscle balance:

1 HIP/LEG EXTENSION

Some participants create an undesirable curve of the lower back with an excessive rear leg lift and exaggerate the problem with a forward body lean.

Figure 2.5

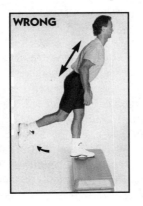

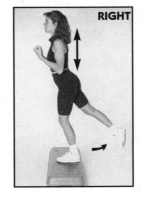

Stand tall on the platform and extend the rear lifting leg **back**, not up.

Figure 2.6

These moves are great exercises for the thighs and buttocks:

2 SIDE STEP-OUT SQUATS

Some participants have a tendency to lean too far out to the side, which places too much stress on the knee.

Figure 2.7

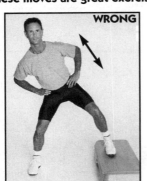

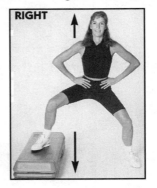

Balance your weight evenly, keeping your center of gravity squarely within your legs.

Figure 2.8

3 STEP-BACK LUNGES FROM PLATFORM

Do not bend too far forward at the hip or have your leg reaching back in a locked-knee position. Also, heel should not be forced to the ground; this position may be too much dorsiflexion of the foot for you.

Figure 2.9

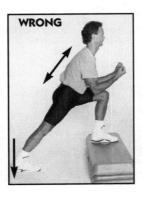

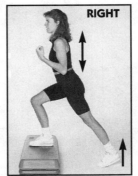

Keep your body weight predominantly over the platform leg, and keep your knee over your toes. The leg reaching back should make floor contact, with your knee slightly flexed. This will help reduce any chance of joint trauma from ground impact. Back heel is raised up off the floor.

Figure 2.10

very strong, whereas the back muscles are relatively weak. All heavy lifting should be done by stabilizing the back in an erect position and making the *legs* provide the necessary power.

Get as close to the object as possible, using a forward-stride position. The object should be in front of you if you are using two hands (e.g., step bench) or beside you if you are using one hand (e.g., luggage). Keep your back straight and your pelvis tucked, and bend at the hips, knees, and ankles to lower your body. Lower directly downward, only as much as necessary.

Both arms should be placed well under or *around the weight center* of the load. Lift vertically upward in a slow, steady movement by extending your leg muscles. Keep the object close to your weight center (Figure 2.11). Reverse the procedure to lower the object.

✢ *Do not* bend over from the hips (head low, buttocks high), as that would make your back muscles lift the load (Figure 2.12).

Correct Carrying

✢ Keep the object close to your weight center.

✢ Separate the load when feasible, and carry half in each hand/arm (Figure 2.13).

SUMMARY

A bench/step training program has many advantages and benefits. The key is that it is a high-intensity exercise that sustains the training zone heart-rate needed to produce the cardiorespiratory training effect. Yet, it is low-impact and safe, as one foot remains on the bench or the ground. Maintaining the safe precautions of selecting the correct bench height, good body positioning and alignment, and variety in technique, to prevent over-use, all work together to establish an exciting new modality variety of aerobics training. You've now taken the first step.

Correct Lifting and Carrying

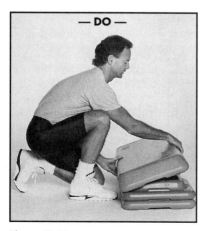

Figure 2.11

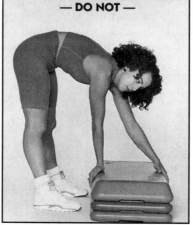

Figure 2.12

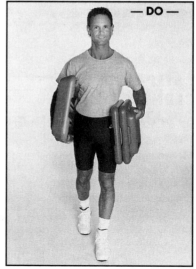

Figure 2.13

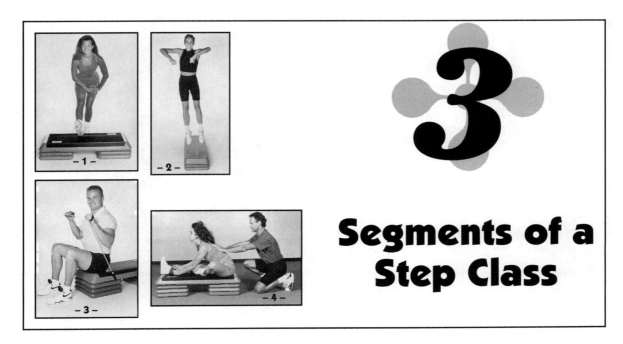

Segments of a Step Class

Step training is an exercise that can significantly improve your cardiovascular fitness. It also promotes a wide variety of other benefits, such as cardiovascular endurance enabling you to perform for longer periods, coordination improvement, and greater strength and flexibility of the skeletal muscles.

An effective step training fitness workout includes four segments: (1) warm-up/stretch, (2) step aerobics, (3) strength training/isolation exercises, and (4) cool-down, flexibility, and relaxation. When these four segments are incorporated into your step training program, you can achieve overall physical fitness. Using the following principles and guidelines for each segment will help to achieve the results you desire.[1, 2, 3, 4, 5]

WARM-UP SEGMENT

The warm-up begins with active, low-level, rhythmic, limbering, standing, range-of-motion types of exercises that raise the body's core temperature slightly, initiate muscular movements, and prepare you for more strenuous moves to come. Involve the step-bench by performing moves that integrate use of both the floor and the bench. Example: Perform bench step taps, with bicep curls (Figure 3.1). Use low-impact moves that allow you to adjust to the height and contour of the bench, such as stepping up and down at half the tempo, marching on top of the bench, or straddling the bench and alternating tapping on top of the bench (Figure 3.2). The time-frame is approximately 5 minutes.

After the muscles, tendons, ligaments, and joints are loose and pliable, exercise takes the form of slow, sustained, static stretching. Static stretching, probably the most popular, easiest, and safest form of stretching, involves gradually stretching a muscle or muscle group to the point of limitation, then holding that position for approximately 15 seconds. The stretch is repeated to the opposite side. Several repetitions of each stretch are performed. Static stretching is recommended when muscles are *warm* (after the initial active phase of the warm-up and later after intense physical activity).

Stretch all major muscles from head to toe (Figures 3.3–3.5), with special consideration for

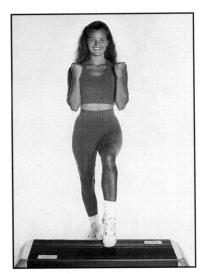

Figure 3.1 Bench step taps, with bicep curls.

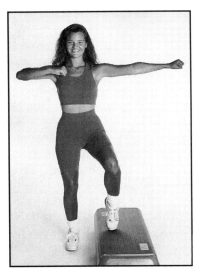

Figure 3.2 Alternate tapping on top, from the straddle position.

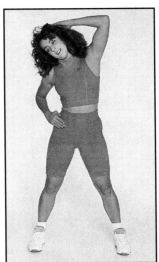

Figure 3.3 Drop head to the side and press.

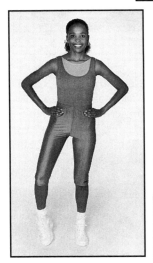

Figure 3.4 Ankle stretching, circling out.

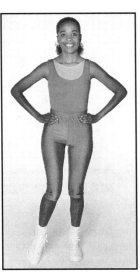

Figure 3.5 Ankle stretching, circling in.

the major muscle groups in the legs, such as the thighs, hips, and calves, as step training is lower body intensive. When step training, the bench can be used as a fixed object to enhance stretching (Figures 3.6–3.9).[6]

BREATHING TECHNIQUE

Breathe continuously. Your entire system, especially your working muscles, constantly need oxygen. Holding your breath and turning red is never an appropriate way to exercise. While performing the warm-up and cool-down stretching (or any strengthening exercise), exhale when you stretch, by puckering your lips and breathing out, and inhale when you relax your muscles.

Cue yourself: "Breathe out and stretch"; "breathe in and relax."

The time-frame for the warm-up stretching segment is approximately 5 minutes.

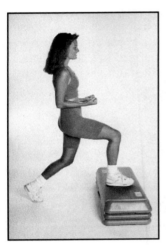

Figure 3.6 Hip flexors — facing the bench.

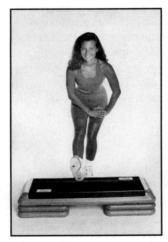

Figure 3.8 Hamstring stretch — facing the bench.

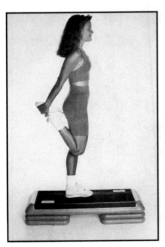

Figure 3.7 Quadricep stretch — standing on the bench.

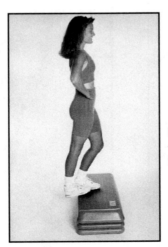

Figure 3.9 Calf stretch — standing on top of the bench.

⋅⊱
STEP AEROBICS SEGMENT

The aerobics segment can be subdivided into sections, each focusing on the impact you perform in relation to the heart rate intensity you are building, sustaining, or lowering, and according to which phase of the hour you're in. Heart rate should be monitored at least twice during the 30–40 minute segment.

This segment begins with the pre-aerobic phase, a progressive transition from the warm-up into the high-intensity aerobic phase. Example: Perform basic steps with a variety of arm movements (Figure 3.10). Pre-aerobic moves are performed at a moderate tempo to gradually increase the body's temperature and heart rate.

During the aerobic segment, the intensity of the exercises (measured as heart rate BPM) should increase gradually to your fitness level. Vary your movements to maintain interest level, ensure safety, and effectively work as many muscles as possible. Begin by coordinating both the arms and the legs (Figures 3.11–3.12), then build more difficult movement patterns (Figure 3.13–3.14).

Finally, to provide a transition between the vigorous aerobic work and the anaerobic strength training segment of the workout, the heart rate must be gradually brought back down to the normal (pre-exercise) heart rate. This helps prevent a build-up of lactic acid (metabolic waste product) and keeps the blood from pooling in the lower extremities. Like the pre-aerobic phase, the post-aerobic cool-down is performed at a slower tempo and consists of lower range-of-motion movements (Figure 3.15).

⋅⊱
Progressing Safely Through the Step Aerobics Segment

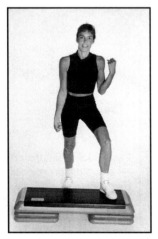

Figure 3.10 V-step with bicep curl.

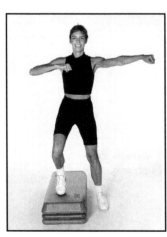

Figure 3.11

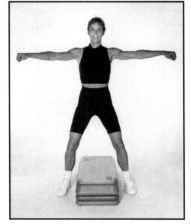

Figure 3.12
Straddle down, arms follow.

❖
Progressing Safely Through the Step Aerobics Segment

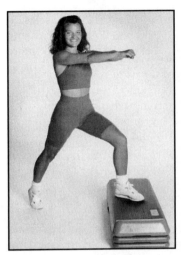

Figures 3.13 Lunge right.

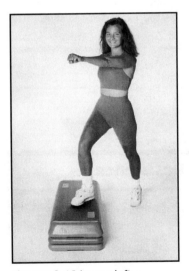

Figures 3.14 Lunge left.

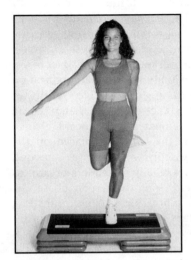

Figure 3.15 Post-aerobic cool down: Hamstring curl touch heel in back.

❖

ISOLATION EXERCISES/ STRENGTH TRAINING SEGMENT

During vigorous aerobics, all muscles of the body are strengthened. The strength segment (included within an aerobics workout focusing on the strength development of isolated muscle groups) follows the aerobics workout but comes before the final cool-down, flexibility training, and relaxation segment. The reasoning is simple. With an increase in the resistance (weight) that must be applied to any movement for significant change (training) to occur, the workload placed on the heart, lungs, and vascular system also increases. An individual is more readily placed in a breathless "oxygen-debt" state. During the aerobic phase, the goal is *not* to be in a breathless state but, instead, in a breathe-easy state, steadily pacing the intensity.

The isolation exercises/strength training segment focuses on specific muscle groups in a steady, controlled manner, (which tends to sustain proper body postural alignment), *concentrating on areas not adequately worked during the aerobic segment*. In contrast to step aerobics, which is lower body intensive, this segment works the muscles in the upper body and the abdominals, in two or three sets of 8 to 12 repetitions. This prescription is for all muscle groups except the abdominals. Repetitions can be increased to 15–30 for each of the two sets.

To incorporate variety into the strength training segment, different forms of resistance, such as hand-held weights, resistance bands, and tubing, can be used. Sample strength/bench exercises that work isolated muscle groups are: for the chest, push-ups (Figure 3.16) and bent-arm chest crossover (Figures 3.17 and 3.18); for the arms and shoulders, short-lever bicep curls (Figure 3.19) and long-lever lateral raises (Figure 3.20); for the abdomen, curl-up variations (Figure 3.21); and for the buttocks, squats (Figure 3.22).

These exercises are done to more quickly define, tone, shape, and make more dense (thicken) the muscle fibers. They also allow longer periods of work during the exercise program and later in daily work tasks. Chapter 6 provides principles, guidelines, and suggested exercises for safe, effective strength training.

❖

Strength Training Segment Using a Variety of Resistance

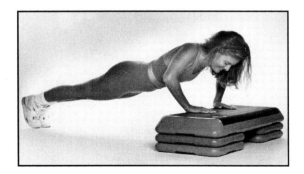

Figure 3.16 (Chest) Push-up on the bench (your weight).

✢
Strength Training Segment Using a Variety of Resistance

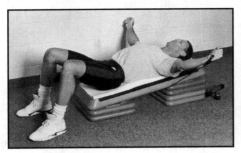

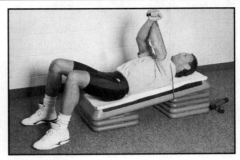

Figure 3.17   **Figure 3.18**
(Chest) Bent Arm Chest Cross-Over (tubing).

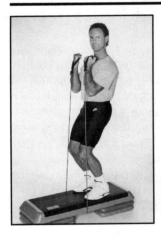

Figure 3.19 (Arms & Shoulders) Short-lever bicep curls (tubing).

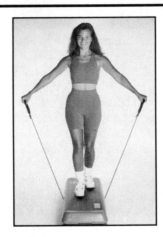

Figure 3.20 (Arms & Shoulders) Long-lever lateral raises (tubing).

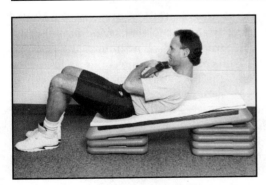

Figure 3.21 (Abdominals) Gravity-Assisted Curl-Up (incline bench and 1-4 lb. weights).

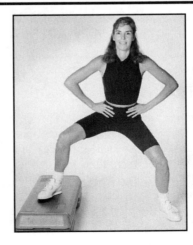

Figure 3.22 (Buttocks) Squats (bench).

∻

COOL-DOWN, FLEXIBILITY, AND RELAXATION SEGMENT

The purpose of a cool-down segment in the workout is to give the body time to readjust to the pre-activity state. This eases the gradual process of returning the large quantity of blood now in the working muscles (primarily in the arms and legs) back toward the vital organs in the head and trunk. Abruptly stopping a highly strenuous activity session may cause the blood (primarily in the legs) to "pool" or stay in the extremities, because the veins of the legs are not being forcefully squeezed now by strenuously working leg muscles. This pooling can cause cramping, nausea, dizziness, and fainting, as the needed quantity of oxygen and blood is not being delivered to the brain and other vital organs.

The ability to recover from exertion usually determines the length of cool-down. A minimum of 5 to 10 minutes is essential, however, (a) to curtail profuse sweating, and (b) to lower the heart rate to below 120 beats per minute. These are two visible signs to monitor and achieve before concluding the exercise hour.

You'll begin the cooling down process by slowing down all large-muscle activity. Tapering off the activity level can be done in various ways, such as performing slow-tempo, low-impact aerobics moves (Figure 3.23). This segment begins the transition between the vigorous bench/strength activity just completed, and the flexibility training and relaxation performed last.

FLEXIBILITY TRAINING

Flexibility training, or *stretching*, is widely accepted as an effective means of increasing joint mobility, improving exercise performance, and reducing injuries.[7] Proper technique is essential, for the risks of injury may be significant if stretches are performed incorrectly.

Flexibility refers to the *range-of-motion of a given joint and its corresponding muscle groups.*

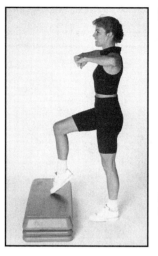

Step Tap

Figure 3.23 Cool-down with a Step Tap.

It is genetically influenced and highly specific and varies from joint to joint within an individual. When repeatedly stretched, muscle can be lengthened by approximately 20 percent[8]; tendons can increase in length only about 2 to 3 percent.

Stretching programs follow the principle of specific adaptation to imposed demands (SAID), which states that an individual must slowly and progressively stretch the soft tissues around a joint to and slightly beyond the point of limitation but not to the point of tearing.

Two Methods of Stretching

At present, the two most widely accepted methods of stretching for improving flexibility are static and proprioceptive neuromuscular facilitatory (PNF) techniques. Both techniques follow the philosophy that flexibility is increased and risk of injury is prevented when the muscle being stretched is as relaxed as possible.

Static stretching is slow, active stretching, and the position is held at the joint extremes. The technique for executing stretching efficiently and safely is to gently ease into a controlled, stretched position and hold it as you gently press (Figure 3.24). Push or press to the point of tightness, "stretch pull" (a tight feeling but not a pain) so you

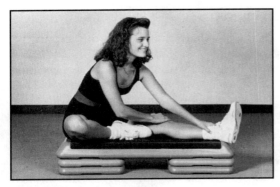

Figure 3.24 Static stretching.

feel the muscle working. Continue to stretch a little beyond this point without any motion. Mentally, then relax your mind and hold the position for approximately 15 seconds, allowing the muscle to also relax and feel heavier.[9] Continue to relax and slowly withdraw the stretch. The same stretching on the opposite side of the body always follows.

At present, static stretching is considered to be one of the most effective methods of increasing flexibility, and research has shown that significant gains can be achieved with a training program of static stretching exercises. This type of continuous, long stretching produces greater flexibility with less possibility of injury, probably because it stretches the muscles under controlled conditions.

PNF stretching, in which muscles are stretched progressively with intermittent isometric contractions, are also effective in increasing flexibility and are used, like static stretches, when the muscles are warm. Two of the most commonly used modified PNF stretches are:

❖ *Contract-relax technique:* In phase one, the exerciser does a 5- to 6-second maximum voluntary contraction in the muscle to be stretched. The contraction is isometric because any motion is resisted. In phase two, the previously contracted muscle is relaxed, then stretched.

❖ *Agonist contract-relax technique*: In phase one, the exerciser maximally contracts the muscle opposite the muscle to be stretched against

resistance (a partner, the floor, or other immovable object) for 5 to 6 seconds. In phase two, the agonist muscle is relaxed and the antagonist muscle is stretched.[10]

An example of a forward PNF contract-relax exercise for the hamstrings and spinal extensors, shown in Figure 3.25, is performed with a partner's assistance. The position and actions are detailed.

❖ *Position*: In a modified hurdler stretch position, the performing partner leans forward to the point of limitation while keeping the back straight and the toes of the extended leg facing upward to correctly stretch the hamstrings.

❖ *Action*: To begin the action, the performer pushes her back against her partner (contracting the spinal extensors) and pushes the extended leg against the floor (contracting the hamstrings) for a 6-second isometric contraction. The partner gently but firmly resists any movement.

❖ *Action*: After releasing the contraction, the performer stretches to a new point of limitation, holding a static stretch for 12 seconds or more while the partner maintains a light pressure on the performer's back.

Research has shown that *both* static and PNF techniques for stretching are effective. Each can be used successfully to enhance flexibility.

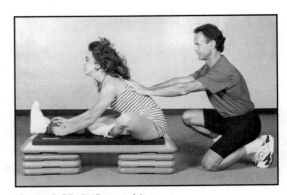

Figure 3.25 PNF stretching.

TIME TO STRETCH

Stretching to increase flexibility and range of motion is crucial now. It is a time when the muscles are warm (full of blood, oxygen, and nutrients) and the joints are pliable from vigorous exercise. Take full advantage of the next 5 to 10 minutes to static or PNF stretch (Figures 3.26–3.29).

STATIC STRETCHING WITH RELAXATION

Relaxation techniques complete the total physical fitness hour and can begin during the stretching phase (Figure 3.30), to realize greater flexibility gains, and continue when stretching is completed, upon the absence of muscle tension throughout the body (Figure 3.31).

The participant focuses on three key factors:

✛ Mental images you are constructing.

✛ Self-talk accompanying each stretch and release (or contract-relax, according to which technique you use).

✛ The mechanics of your breathing pattern.

The mental images now match the accompanying self-talk. The muscles being isolated and stretched are pictured and affirmed as becoming "wider, and longer, warmer and heavier."

Your breathing pattern is sequenced with these pictures and affirmations. An eight-count deep breath starts the whole procedure and is initiated from deep down in the diaphragm area and inhaled through the nose. This deep breath is held several seconds (up to 8). As you slowly exhale through pursed lips, formulate the pictures and affirmations: "wider-longer-warmer-heavier" . . . "wider-longer-warmer-heavier." Take about 16 seconds to slowly exhale and static stretch with these pictures and affirmations. Finally, as the stretch is slowly released and the muscle relaxed, begin another deep eight-count inhalation.

To match pictures and affirmations with the PNF stretching, mentally take apart the muscular actions and the time-frame suggested for each portion. Do exhalation breathing during the contractions.

A complete program of relaxation techniques is presented in Chapter 7 to finalize your total physical fitness workout hour.

– CLASS NOTES –

❖ Flexibility Training

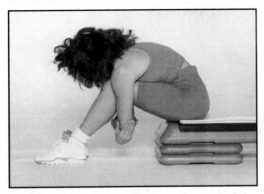

Figure 3.26. Back Stretch. Sit on the end of the bench with your feet together on the floor. Bend over, resting your chest on thighs. Reach under legs with arms, grasp the opposite elbow, and pull both elbows together. Hold.

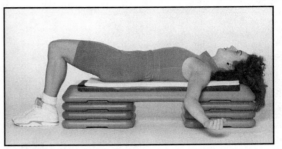

Figure 3.27. Pectoral Stretch. Lie down on the platform with head and buttocks both comfortably on bench. Press the low back into the bench and place arms out wide to the sides, shoulder level, palms up. Relax arms as their weight falls toward the floor. Hold.

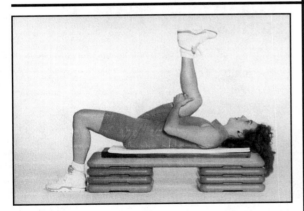

Figure 3.28. Hamstring Stretch. Still lying on the bench, extend the L leg straight out along the platform and place foot flat on floor. Grasp behind the R thigh and gently pull the R leg toward the chest. Hold.

Ankle Circling: During the hamstring stretch, slowly circle the foot in all directions. Alternate with L leg and foot.

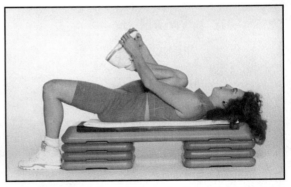

Figure 3.29. Achilles/Calf Stretch. From the hamstring stretch, pull R knee to chest. Grasp R toes with the hands, and gently pull. Hold. Alternate with L leg and foot.

❖
Static Stretching With Relaxation

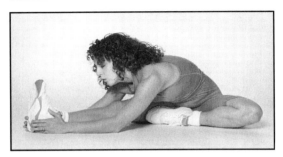

Figure 3.30. Relaxation can begin during the static stretching.

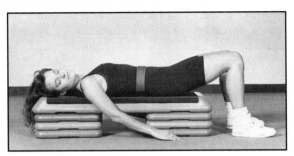

Figure 3.31. Continue when stretching is completed.

❖
STEP AEROBIC PROGRAM SEGMENTS IN REVIEW

The basic principles for the four key segments of a step aerobics program workout session are:

SEGMENT 1: WARM-UP

❖ Active, rhythmic, limbering moves
❖ Slow, standing, static stretching
❖ Proper breathing techniques throughout

SEGMENT 2: STEP AEROBICS

❖ Pre-aerobic/transitional progression from low to high
❖ Aerobic phase
❖ Aerobic cool-down

SEGMENT 3: ISOLATION EXERCISES/STRENGTH TRAINING

❖ Emphasis on isolated muscle groups — chest, arms, abdominals, buttocks
❖ Weights, resistance bands and tubing, and bench exercises added

SEGMENT 4: COOL-DOWN, FLEXIBILITY, AND RELAXATION TECHNIQUES

❖ Gradual cool-down moves
❖ Flexibility training using static and PNF stretching
❖ Relaxation techniques during stretching.

SUMMARY

Adhering to this step aerobics workout format will provide you with a fun, safe, efficient, and complete session. If this type of total physical fitness program is prioritized into your schedule for a minimum of three days per week, you will have an excellent means of initially obtaining, and then maintaining, your fitness for a lifetime.

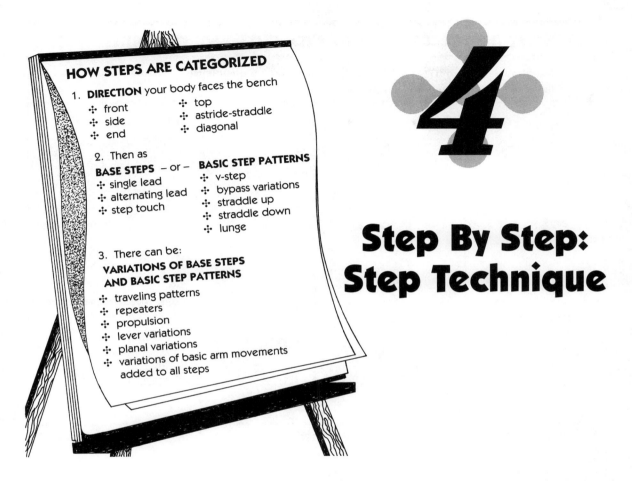

HOW STEPS ARE CATEGORIZED

1. **DIRECTION** your body faces the bench
   - ✛ front
   - ✛ side
   - ✛ end
   - ✛ top
   - ✛ astride-straddle
   - ✛ diagonal

2. Then as

   BASE STEPS – or – **BASIC STEP PATTERNS**
   - ✛ single lead
   - ✛ alternating lead
   - ✛ step touch
   - ✛ v-step
   - ✛ bypass variations
   - ✛ straddle up
   - ✛ straddle down
   - ✛ lunge

3. There can be:

   VARIATIONS OF BASE STEPS AND BASIC STEP PATTERNS
   - ✛ traveling patterns
   - ✛ repeaters
   - ✛ propulsion
   - ✛ lever variations
   - ✛ planal variations
   - ✛ variations of basic arm movements added to all steps

Step By Step: Step Technique

The step aerobic techniques in this chapter represent movement depicting

✛ directional approaches and orientations (your body in relation to the bench)

✛ base steps

✛ basic step patterns

✛ variations possible, using base steps and basic step patterns (see graphic above)

These step techniques are photographed and described by the "mirroring technique" for all *front* views shown (actual left of model is your right). Natural photography is used and described for all *side* and *rear* views. The words and the movements, therefore, are to be performed *exactly* as shown.

If you're following the movements of an instructor, position the bench for maximum visibility.

BENCH/STEP DIRECTIONAL APPROACHES AND ORIENTATIONS[1]

Initial movement onto the bench can begin from one of the following directions — the direction in which your body faces the bench.

From the Front

Facing the bench squarely.

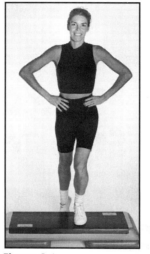

Figure 4.1

From the End

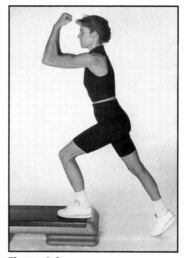

Facing the **end** of the bench, step up and down.

Figure 4.2

From the Side

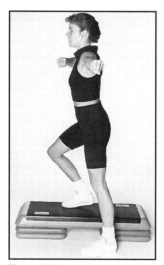

Standing with **your side** next to the bench's **side**, step up with the foot that is closest to the side of the bench.

Standing with **your side** next to the **end** of the bench, step up with the foot that is closest to the side of the bench.

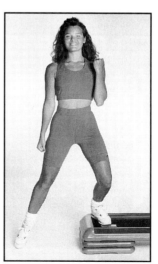

Figure 4.3

Figure 4.4

✛
BENCH/STEP DIRECTIONAL APPROACHES AND ORIENTATIONS

From the Top

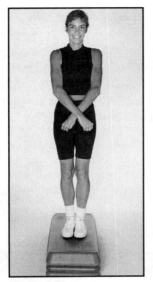

Atop, facing the bench's **end**, with feet together.

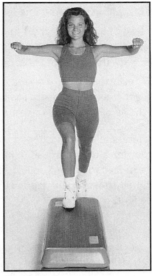

Atop, standing at the **back end of the bench**, step off the back in a forward/backward stride.

Figure 4.5   **Figure 4.6**

Astride/ Straddle

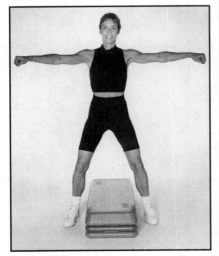

Facing the bench's **end**, standing astride or straddle position, with bench between your feet.

Figure 4.7

Diagonal

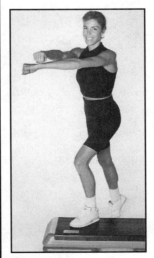

Facing on an **angle** toward the bench's corner; if facing at an angle to the left, step up with the right foot first, and if facing at an angle to the right, step up with the left foot first.

Figure 4.8

BASE STEPS

There are three base steps which may be performed using a variety of directional approaches/ orientations. They are identified as:

⋅⋅⋅ a **single lead step,** in which the **same** foot leads **every 4-count cycle;**

⋅⋅⋅ an **alternate lead step** — the right and left foot both serve as the lead foot **alternately initiating every 4 counts**, requiring a complete cycle for the alternating patterns to take **8 counts** (i.e., both the right foot and then left foot lead a 4-count portion of the cycle);

⋅⋅⋅ a **step touch**, performed by "touching" the *same* toe or heel on the floor or bench or by *alternating* legs. Step touch moves are often used during the warm-up segment to familiarize you with the bench, or as transition moves during the aerobic segment.

For both safety and variety when using single-lead step, 4-count cycle patterns, lead with the right foot for a **maximum of 1 minute**, then change to a left-foot lead. To accomplish this change in lead foot (for single cycle 4-count step patterns), perform a **non-weight-bearing, transitional, hold/touch/ tap/heel** move as the last step of the cycle, initiating the change with that foot.

Within the descriptions, only the moves typed in bold face are shown in the figures.

Single Lead Step

Bench Approach: Front (shown), top, end, and diagonal.

	R	L	R	L	
Right Lead:	**Up**	up	down	**down**	**4 counts**

	L	R	L	R	
Left Lead:	Up	up	down	down	**4 counts**

Arms shown: Long-lever punching on up, up; pull, punch, on the down, down.

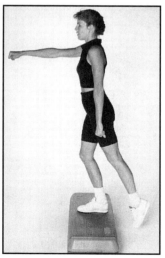

Figure 4.9

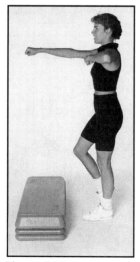

Figure 4.10

BASE STEPS

Alternating Lead Step

You may alternate the lead leg with a bench tap up (on bench) or a floor tap down (on floor).

Bench Approach: Front (shown), top, end, and diagonal.

Bench Tap

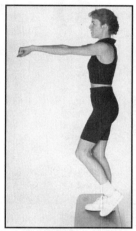

Figure 4.11

R	L	L	R
Up	**bench tap**	down	down

Alternate: Up (L), bench tap (R), down (R), down (L).

8 counts   **Arms shown:** Forward punching.

Floor Tap

R	L	R	L
Up	up	down	**floor tap**

Alternate: Up (L), up (R), down (L), floor tap (R).

8 counts

Arms shown: Opposite-arm long-lever punching; same arm flexing; elbows kept shoulder high.

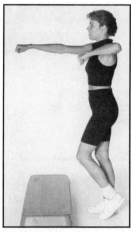

Figure 4.12

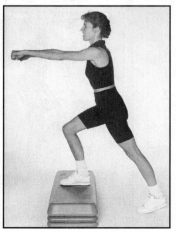

Figure 4.13

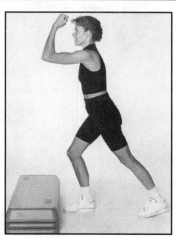

Figure 4.14

Lunge Back

Note: The Floor Tap may also be a non-weight-bearing lunge back.

R	L	R	L
Up	up	down	**down and back**

Alternate, starting with the (L) Up.

8 counts.

Arms shown: Arms punching forward and parallel on up, up; bicep curls keeping elbows still high on the down, down.

BASE STEPS

Step Touch

Bench Approach: Front (shown), top, end, astride.

Step Touch with the Toe

R	R

Bench tap with toe down; repeat with left foot.

4 counts

Arms shown: Elbows shoulder-high, fists together on tap; fists apart on down.

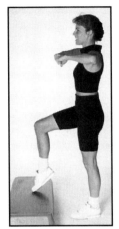

Figure 4.15

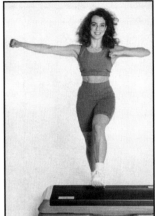

Figure 4.16

Step Touch with the Heel

R	R

Bench tap with heel down; repeat with left foot.

4 counts

Arms shown: Arms extended to the side at shoulder level, alternating punching to the side.

BASIC STEP PATTERNS[2]

Basic step patterns may be performed as single lead steps (4-count pattern) or alternating lead steps (8-count pattern). When performing a **single lead basic step pattern**, the **fourth count** of the cycle is weight-bearing. When executing **alternating lead steps**, there are two options — when the first 3 steps are weight-bearing the 4th is **non-weight bearing** or when the first 3 steps contain a bypass move, the 4th step is **weight-bearing**.

V-Step

Bench Approach: Front.

R	L	R	L
Up-wide	up-wide	**down-center**	down-center

Usually cued: "out" "out" "in" "in".

Arms shown: Same-side single bicep curls.

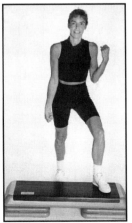

Figure 4.17

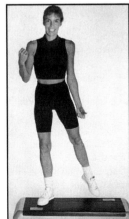

Figure 4.18

BASIC STEP PATTERNS

Bypass Variations (Figure 4.19–4.24)

Bench Approach: Front (shown), side, top, end, diagonal.

Knee up Bypass

L   R
Up, **knee lift** (bypasses the bench and lifts)

    R
down (to floor)

    L
down (to floor)

Arms shown: Initiate from arms fully extended out to the sides, shoulder high with palms up: single short-lever curls on the up and knee lift; return one at a time to the long-lever, shoulder-high initial position on the down, down.

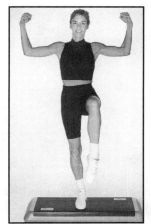

Figure 4.19

Kick Forward Bypass

L   R   R   L
Up **kick forward** down (to floor) down (to floor)

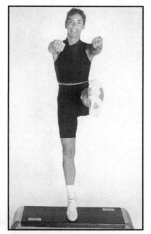

Arms shown: Arms sweep up from sides, together and parallel on up, kick; sweep together and parallel back down to sides on the down, down.

Figure 4.20

Kick Back Bypass

L   R
Up **kick back** (a "**long lever** raising" motion)

    R
down (to floor)

    L
down (to floor)

Arms shown: Initiate from arms fully extended down at sides: Raise same (one) elbow out wide to shoulder high with fist ending at waist, for the up and kick back; lower to initial position at side with each down, down.

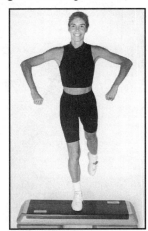

Figure 4.21

Side Leg Lift Bypass

L   R
Up **side leg lift** (a knee pointing forward position),

    R   L
down (to floor)   down (to floor)

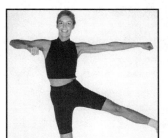

Arms shown: Both arms raised simultaneously to bent-arm lateral raise position for up; same arm (one) extends out to side shoulder high for the side leg lift; extended arm returns to bent-arm lateral raise on the down; both arms lowered simultaneously on the last down.

Figure 4.22

BASIC STEP PATTERNS

Bypass Variations (Figure 4.19–4.24)

Bench Approach: Front (shown), side, top, end, diagonal.

| Adductor Bypass | Hamstring Curl Bypass |

Adductor Bypass

R   L
Up **lift heel to front** (a **short-lever** raising motion)

    L
down (to floor)

    R
down (to floor)

Arms shown: Both arms extend to side at shoulder level when you step up. As the heel lifts to the front, the opposite hand touches the instep; when you step down, the arms lower to the side.

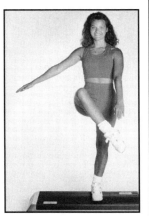

Figure 4.23

Hamstring Curl Bypass

R   L
Up **lift heel to back** (a **short-lever** raising motion)

    L
down (to floor)

    R
down (to floor)

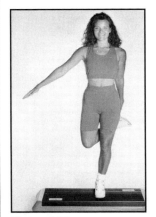

Arms shown: Both arms extend to side at shoulder level when you step up. As the heel lifts to the back, the opposite hand reaches back and touches the heel; when you step down, the arms lower to the side.

Figure 4.24

Straddle Up

Bench Approach: Astride (shown).

R   L
Up **knee lift** (bypasses bench and lifts waist-high),

    L   R
straddle down (to floor)   straddle down (to floor)

Alternate pattern, stepping now up (L) and knee lifting (R), followed by the straddle down, down.

Arms shown: Shoulder high, short-levers, and fists together at center. Opposite arm punches forward on lift.

Note: For variety, try the other bypass moves shown earlier — kick forward, kickback, or side leg lift, incorporating one or more accompanying arm movements that will keep your balance atop the bench. Straddle Up can also be a non-bypass basic step pattern

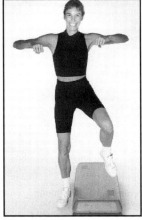

Figure 4.25

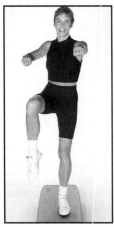

Figure 4.26

Straddle Down

Bench Approach: Top (shown).

R
Straddle Down (on R side of bench)
L
Straddle down (on L side of bench)

R   L
up   up

Arms shown: Shoulder high, short-levers, and fists together at center. Same long-lever arm extends out to side as same leg steps out. One arm at a time returns back in to center on each up, up step.

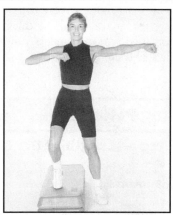

Figure 4.27

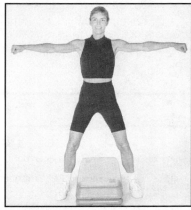

Figure 4.28

Lunge

Bench Approach: Top (shown).	**Bench Approach:** End (shown).

L   L
Touch down side   up
R   R
touch down side   up

Arms shown: When left leg steps to the side, punch the left arm in front at an angle; when right leg steps to the side, punch the right arm in front at an angle.

L   L
Touch down back   up
R   R
touch down back   up

Arms shown: Arms parallel at shoulder level; bicep-curl touch down back; and punch forward on the touch up on bench.

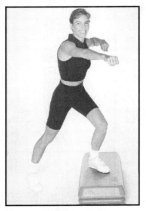

Figure 4.29

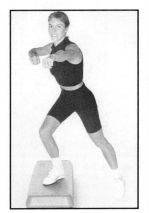

Figure 4.30

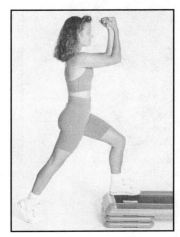

Figure 4.31

VARIATIONS OF BASE STEPS AND BASIC STEP PATTERNS[3]

To add interest and variety to base steps and basic step patterns, a number of variations can be implemented. The following step variations can be categorized as traveling, repeaters, propulsion, lever, and planal. Creative arm movements will also play a significant role in adding variety and interest to the step training workout.

Traveling Patterns (Figure 4.32–4.54)

Turn Step — Length of the Bench

Bench Approach: Side (shown).

Single lead – **4 counts**; Alternating lead – **8 counts**.

L	R	L	R
Up	**body 1/2 turns left and up**	**down**	**tap down**

Arms shown: Shoulder-high alternating punch and pull back.

> **Note** Remember to keep your eyes on the platform. Also, this pattern is shown using natural photography and descriptive words, as it could not be photographed, and therefore described, from a "mirrored" perspective.

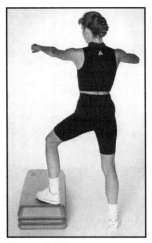
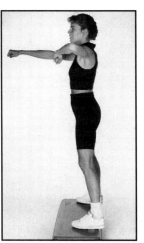
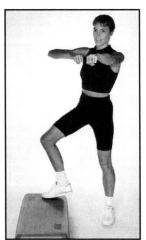
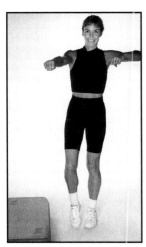

Figure 4.32   **Figure 4.33**   **Figure 4.34**   **Figure 4.35**

Traveling Patterns

Over the Top — Width of the Bench

Bench Approach: Side (shown).

Single lead – **4 counts**; Alternating lead – **8 counts**.

L	R	L	R
Up	**up**	**down on the left side of bench/platform**	**touch down**

Cued: "up", "over", "down", "tap".

> **Note:** For variety on the **fourth** step, instead of tapping the floor: touch heel on the bench; knee up; or kick front.

Arms shown: Elbows pointing skyward and shoulder high, with arms wide open on the first, third, fifth, and seventh steps; arms low and crossed in front on even-numbered steps.

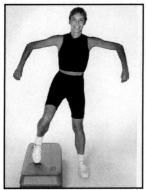
Figure 4.36

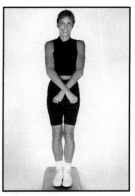
Figure 4.37

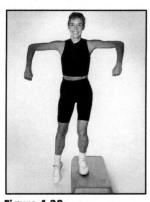
Figure 4.38

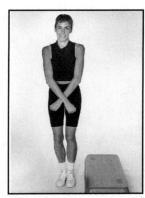
Figure 4.39

Across the Top — Length of the Bench

Bench Approach: End (shown).

Single lead – **4 counts**; Alternating lead – **8 counts.**

R	L	R	L
Up	**up**	**down on the right side of bench**	**touch down**

Cued: "up", "across", "down", "tap".

Arms shown: Arms at shoulder level; when legs are apart, arms are straight out to the side; bend arms into the chest when feet are togther.

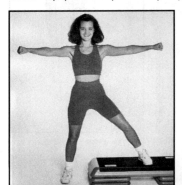
Figure 4.40

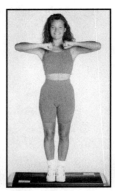
Figure 4.41

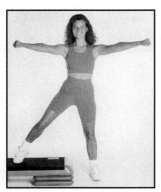
Figure 4.42

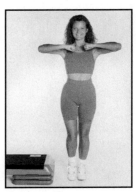
Figure 4.43

Traveling Patterns

Diagonal to Diagonal

Bench Approach: Diagonal (shown).

Alternating lead step – **8 counts.**

  L   R   R   L

Up knee lift   down   down turning body on diagonal facing left corner

> **Note:** For variety on second and sixth steps, use any bypass move (knee, kick front/back, side leg lift, hamstring curl, adductor).

Arms shown: Arms at shoulder level, row position, punch the opposite arm forward as the knee comes up, pull-punch in on down, and both arms punch forward when the body turns to the diagonal.

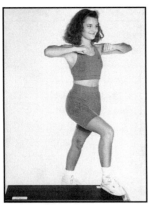

Figure 4.44

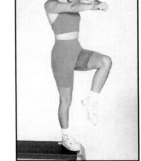

Figure 4.45

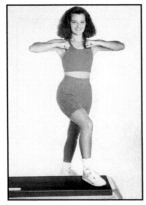

Figure 4.46

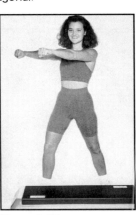

Figure 4.47

Inside End to Outside End

Bench Approach: Side (shown).

Single lead step – **4 counts.**

    L   R   L   R

Up-forward   up   down-forward   down

Cued: "up", "to the middle", "down", "tap".

Arms shown:
Arms to the side at shoulder level, and angled in the direction the body is traveling.

> **Note:** Since you never approach the bench with your back to it, the next steps must use either the close end of the bench, or all floor patterns, to re-align your body so that you have your front or your side facing the bench.

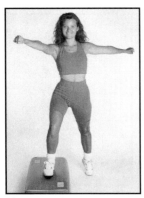

Figure 4.48

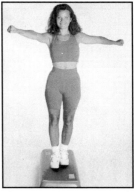

Figure 4.49

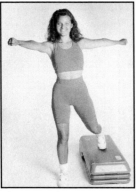

Figure 4.50

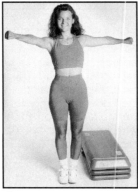

Figure 4.51

Traveling Patterns

Around The Corner

Bench Approach: Side (shown).

Single lead step, 3 cycles each – **4 counts.**

R	L	L	R
Up	**side leg lift**	down (to floor)	tap (on floor)

> **Note:** This variation shows natural photography, since it is a traveling sequence, that can't be mirrored.

Repeat from the **end** (Figure 4.53) and on the **other side** (Figure 4.54) of the bench.

Arms shown: Both arms raised to the side when the leg lifts to the side, and lowered when stepping down to the floor.

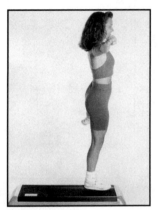

Figure 4.52

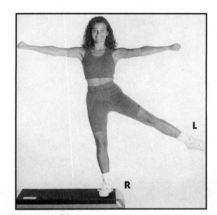

Figure 4.53

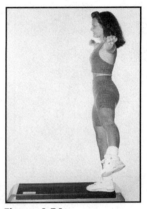

Figure 4.54

Repeaters

This step may be a single or an alternating lead step; however, keep the number of repeaters limited to maximum of 4. A repeater is when any **non-weight-bearing phase of a move is repeated.**

For example: Using a diagonal front approach, **step up (L)**, **tap up (R)**, **tap down and back (R)**, tap up (R), tap down and back (R), tap up (R), step down (R), step down (L) and turn to face the other corner. Alternate stepping up (R) and tapping (L).

> **Note:** For variety, instead of taps use knee lifts, forward kicks, kick backs, side leg lifts, etc.

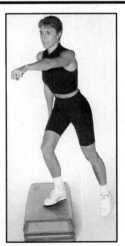

Figure 4.55

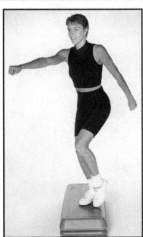

Figure 4.56

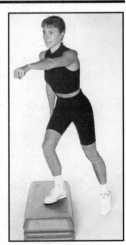

Figure 4.57

Propulsion Steps

Both feet push off the ground or bench, exchanging positions during the airborne phase of the pattern. Propulsion steps are commonly used with lunge steps. A sample propulsion step pattern is shown in Figures 4.58 and 4.59.

Propulsion moves also may be used when performing bypass or traveling moves by adding a hop or pushing off the foot on the bench (Figures 4.60 and 4.61).

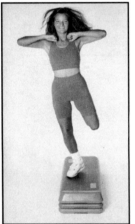 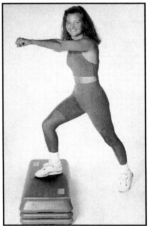 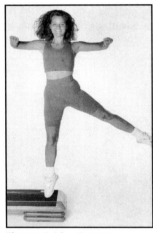 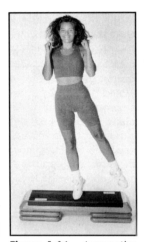

Figure 4.58   **Figure 4.59**   **Figure 4.60**   Bypass.   **Figure 4.61**   Across the
                        Propulsion lunge.   top.

Lever Variations

Lever refers to the joint that initiates the movement. Thus, arm or leg movements may be classified as long- or short-lever movements and can be varied as such. Short-lever moves include knee lifts and bicep curls (Figure 4.62), and long-lever moves include kicks and deltoid raises (Figure 4.63).

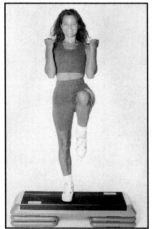 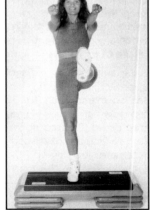

Figure 4.62   Short-levers.   **Figure 4.63**   Long-levers.

Planal Variations

The body can be divided into three different planes: frontal, transverse, and sagittal (Figure 4.64). As an element of variation, planal changes refer to the space in which the arms and/or legs are moving around the body.[4] One way to modify a bypass move, such as a kick front or knee lift in the **frontal plane** (Figures 4.65 and 4.66), would be with a bypass side leg lift or a propulsion lunge in the **sagittal plane** (Figures 4.67 and 4.68). To vary a move in the **transverse plane**, simply keep the same leg movement and vary the arms, or keep the same arm movement and vary the legs.

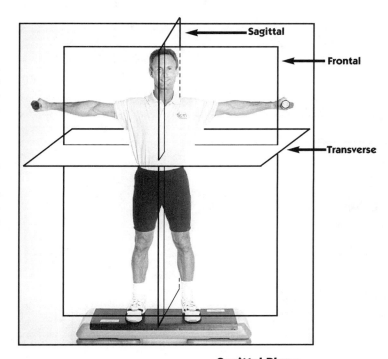

Figure 4.64

Frontal Plane

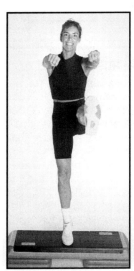

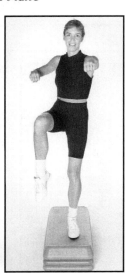

Sagittal Plane

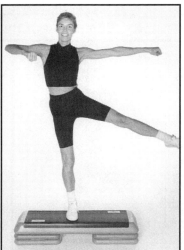

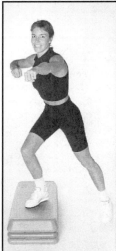

Figure 4.65

Figure 4.66

Figure 4.67

Figure 4.68

VARIATIONS OF BASE STEPS AND BASIC STEP PATTERNS

Variations of Basic Arm Movements

Varying the arm movements adds *significantly* to the variety of your work-out. Before adding any arm movements, however, be sure you are comfortable with the base steps and basic step patterns, and then progress gradually with the easier and less intense versions of the following variations. When the steps are safely mastered, add the more difficult and intense arm movements.

Bilateral / Unilateral

EASY

Bilateral moves refer to movements that are performed in unison or both arms doing the same action.

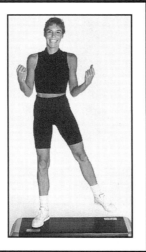

Figure 4.69

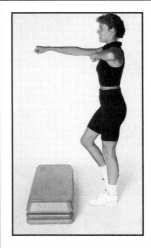

MORE DIFFICULT

Unilateral refers to performing moves in which each arm or leg is doing something different.

Figure 4.70

Complementary / Opposition

EASY

Complementary moves refer to coordinating arm and leg movements. For example, when the left leg moves the left arm moves, and when the right leg moves the right arm moves.

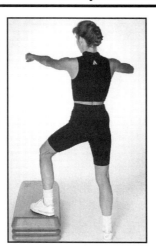

Figure 4.71

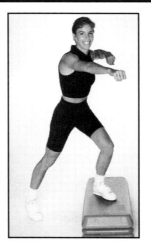

MORE DIFFICULT

Opposition moves are naturally flowing and help you maintain balance but psychologically are usually more challenging when step training. An opposition move is one in which the left arm moves with the right leg and the right arm moves with the left leg.

Figure 4.72

VARIATIONS OF BASE STEPS AND BASIC STEP PATTERNS

Low-/Middle-/Upper-Range Arm Movements

Start with the less intense, low-range motions (elbows kept low, near your waist), and gradually incorporate more intense, middle-range motions (elbows are chest-to-shoulder high), and then the highly intense upper-range arm movements (elbows are at and above shoulder level).

Low-Range (Elbow) Arm Movements

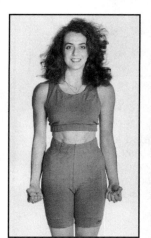 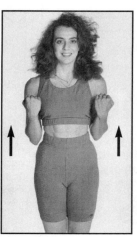 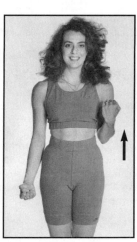

BICEP CURLS

With elbows **fixed** at the sides, **palms up** (Figure 4.73), flex both elbows, forearms moving toward shoulders (Figure 4.74). For **Alternating Bicep Curls**, alternate the right and left forearms (Figure 4.75).

Figure 4.73   **Figure 4.74**   **Figure 4.75**

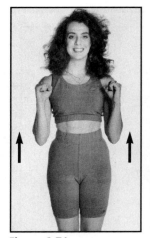 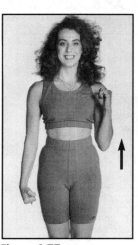

HAMMER CURLS

With elbows **fixed** at the sides and **palms facing** each other, flex both elbows, forearms toward the shoulders (Figure 4.76). For **Alternating Hammer Curls**, alternate the right and left forearms (Figure 4.77).

Figure 4.76   **Figure 4.77**

Low-Range (Elbow) Arm Movements

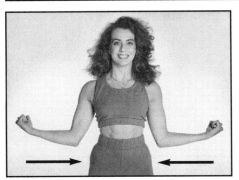

Figure 4.78

LOW WIDE 'N CROSS

With the elbows at the sides and forearms wide (Figure 4.78), criss-cross the arms at waist level in front of the body, keeping palms up. By rotating both elbows forward, **Low Punches** can be performed, by extending both elbows forward, away from the body (palms still up), or **Alternating Low Punches** by extending one forearm at a time.

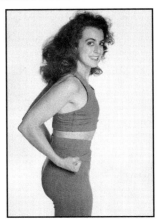

Figure 4.79

ROW LOW

Begin with forearms (only) extended in front of body, waist-level. Pull the elbows backward (Figure 4.79) until fists are next to the waist; return to starting position.

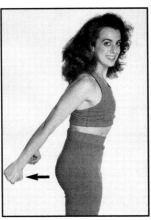

Figure 4.80

TRICEP KICK BACKS

With the elbows **fixed** behind the shoulders and fists next to sides (Figure 4.79), extend both elbows, forearms moving backward (Figure 4.80). For **Alternating Tricep Kick Backs**, alternate right and left arms. Palms can face up/in/down.

Mid-Range Arm Movements

CRISS-CROSSOVER

Keeping elbows at chest height, criss-cross the arms over each other, palms facing down (Figure 4.81). Alternate the arm that crosses over the top, for each repetition (Figure 4.82).

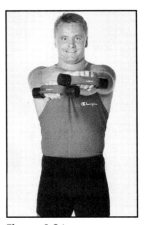

Figure 4.81

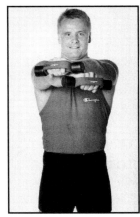

Figure 4.82

Mid-Range Arm Movements

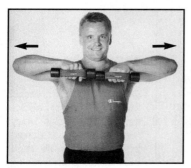

Figure 4.83

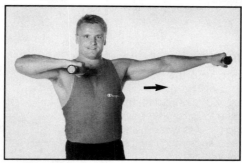

Figure 4.84

DOUBLE AND SINGLE SIDE-OUT

Begin with fists under chin at shoulder level, palms down, elbows directly out (Figure 4.83). Extend both arms wide out to the sides, keeping elbows at shoulder height. Pull the fists back into the chin. For **Single Side-Outs**, alternate the right and left arms (Figure 4.84).

FRONT SHOULDER RAISES

Begin with the palms together in front of the thighs. Keeping elbows soft, raise both arms straight up to the front to shoulder level, palms down (Figure 4.85). Alternate right and left arms, for **Alternating Front Shoulder Raise** (Figure 4.86).

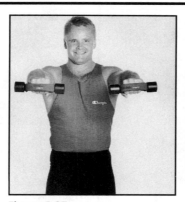

Figure 4.85

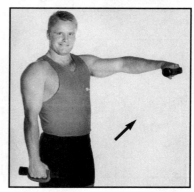

Figure 4.86

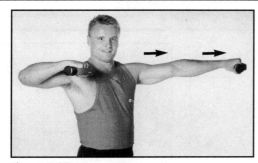

Figure 4.87

SHOULDER PUNCH

Start with the hands lightly resting on the shoulders. Extend one arm forward (Figure 4.87), **or** diagonally across the body, at shoulder height. Pull back and return to shoulder.

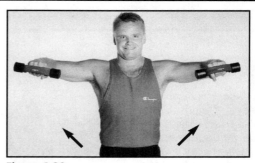

Figure 4.88

SIDE LATERAL RAISE

Start with the fists together in front of the thighs. Lift arms up and out wide, palms facing down, always leading with the elbows, keeping them slightly bent (Figure 4.88).

Mid-Range Arm Movements

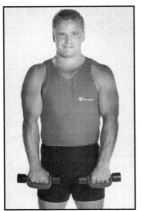

Figure 4.89

UPRIGHT ROW
Begin with the palms in front of the thighs (Figure 4.89). Keeping the fists close to the body and elbows wide, raise the hands up to chin (Figure 4.90).

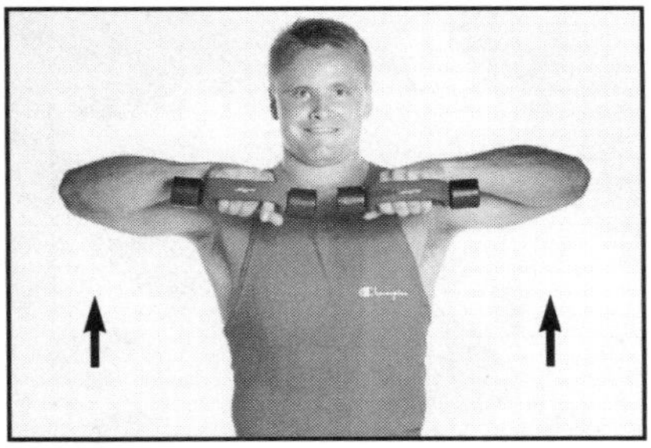

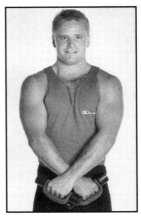

Figure 4.91

CROSS AND LATERAL RAISE
Begin with arms crossed low in front of abdomen, palms facing body (Figure 4.91). Uncross palms and laterally raise elbows up pointing skyward to shoulder height, keeping arms wide open (Figure 4.92).

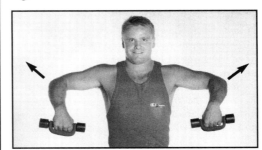

Figure 4.90

Figure 4.92

Upper-Range Arm Movements

SIDE-L
Begin with fists resting on shoulders (Figure 4.93). Simultaneously extend one arm straight out to side at shoulder height while extending the other arm upward above the head (Figure 4.94). Pull both fists back to shoulders and repeat, other direction.

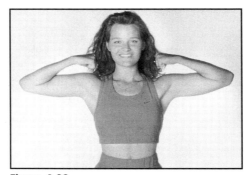

Figure 4.93

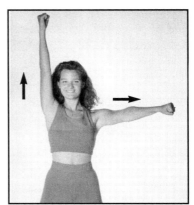

Figure 4.94

Upper-Range Arm Movements

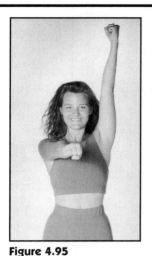

Figure 4.95

FRONT-L

Start with fists resting on shoulders (see Figure 4.93). Simultaneously extend one arm straight out in front of you, shoulder height, while extending other arm upward above the head (Figure 4.95). Pull both fists back to shoulders and repeat, other direction.

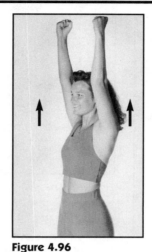

Figure 4.96

OVERHEAD PRESS

Start with fists resting on shoulders (see Figure 4.93). With palms facing, extend arms upward over head, keeping elbows close to ears (Figure 4.96). For **Alternating Overhead Press**, alternate the right and left arms.

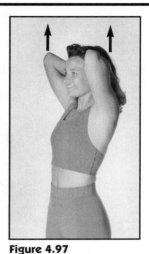

Figure 4.97

TRICEPS EXTENSION

Begin with elbows fixed high, near ears, and fists on shoulders (Figure 4.97). With palms facing, extend arms high and parallel overhead (see Figure 4.96).

SLICE

Begin with fists facing and resting on shoulders, elbows low at sides (Figure 4.98). Simultaneously extend one arm upward straight above head while extending the other arm downward, along side of the leg (Figure 4.99). Pull both fists back to shoulders, and repeat with other side high/low.

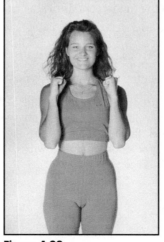

Figure 4.98

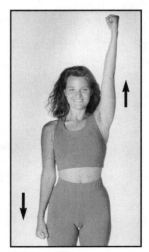

Figure 4.99

Upper-Range Arm Movements

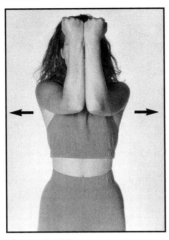

Figure 4.100

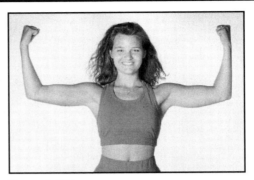

Figure 4.101

BUTTERFLIES

Begin with fists and forearms together and parallel in front of face, elbows pointing down (Figure 4.100). Keeping elbows shoulder-high, open them wide and out to the sides (Figure 4.101).

SUMMARY — STEP TRAINING TECHNIQUES

Techniques illustrating the fundamentals of step training presented here include:

❖ Methods to directionally approach the bench

❖ The base steps and basic step patterns

❖ Techniques for adding variety to the basic step movements

As you advance in your fitness and stepping skills, adding variety will become your next challenge, not only by developing more intricate foot patterns but also by adding many powerful arm movements, taken primarily from strength training principles. Chapter 5, detailing the principles of choreography, will challenge your creative potential for putting unique possibilities together.

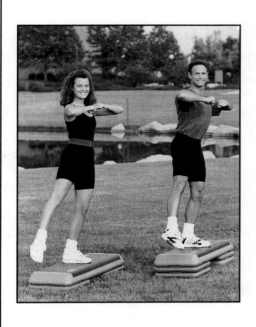

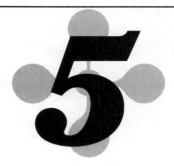

Step to the Beat: Designing and Applying Choreography

Choreography is defined as the art of designing or planning movements.[1] Step training involves stepping on, off, over, and around the bench while doing a series of choreographed movements to music. Outside, inside, in a class setting with a group, on a trip, alone at home — the location is your choice. The moves range from simple base steps to more complex basic step patterns. Once the base steps and basic step patterns are mastered, they may be put together to create a variety of challenging patterns and combinations.

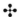

RECIPE FOR SUCCESS

Choreographing aerobic step training can be compared metaphorically to making a classic, time-honored recipe. A recipe requires three things to achieve the same excellent results that can be duplicated again and again by anyone: (1) the *ingredients* (key components), (2) the *amounts* of each ingredient, and (3) the *order* in

which they are best used. Choreography, too, requires key ingredients or basic components for a balanced program, the amounts or numbers of movement possibilities and repetitions of those moves, and the order of their importance (methodology). This constitutes the recipe or blueprint for consistent success. With an understanding of these three factors (*ingredients/amounts/order*), you can become the creative source of your own personal program, or for use when you are placed in the leadership role of directing others.

BALANCED CHOREOGRAPHY

In step training, exercise movements are planned around these three key ingredients:[2]

+ *Biomechanical safety*, to avoid injuries;

+ *Physiological considerations*, to consistently achieve the overall training effect and other individual fitness goals;

∴ *Psychological considerations*, to achieve short-term, present-moment enjoyment and long-term enjoyment for program adherence.

These ingredients must be factored into your planning and then expressed, moment-by-moment, as directed creative movement.

TRANSITIONS

Transition means the flow of one movement to the next. When designing combinations and patterns, transitions are necessary to develop balanced choreography. In step training, as in aerobics, some moves easily follow one another. Table 5.1 lists base moves and basic step patterns that "go together."[3]

COMBINING MOVEMENTS

The two basic ways to put individual step training moves together are linear progressions and repeating progressions. Each can meet the challenge of keeping fun in your fitness pursuits.

LINEAR PROGRESSIONS

Linear movements consist of consecutive repetitions — one following another, then another,

and so on. Linear progressions are used to introduce new moves, add variations, gradually increase intensity, and "build" sequences.[4]

Single-Skill Sequence

Start with one base move or basic step pattern and change one element at a time. For example, using an alternating lead turn-step (length of the bench) (Figures 4.32–4.35), perform four 8-count cycles (32 counts). Then change one element (arms, legs, intensity) at a time. As possibilities for change, instead of a **tap down** (Figure 5.1), perform a **lunge back** (Figure 5.2), a **knee up** (Figure 5.3), or a **chest press** (Figure 5.4).

Begin by performing four 8-count cycles of each element, then break it down from four to two to one 8-count cycle.

REPEATING PROGRESSIONS

The second way of putting moves together is a building block method called repeating progressions. These are a series of single-skill movements combined to form a particular combination. One or more of these movement combinations repeat during a cycle. By beginning with a base step move or basic step pattern, then adding another and putting them together, you create a multiple-skill pattern combination consisting of two, three, four, or more step patterns in a sequence.

Table 5.1

Base Step to:	Knee Up to:	Tap Step to:	Turn Step to:	Over the Top to:	Straddle Down to:	Straddle Up to:
knee up	traveling knee up	knee up	tap down	tap down	over the top	repeaters
tap up	base step	traveling knee up	over the top	turn step	lunge	tap down
v-step	repeaters	turn step	straddle down		tap ups	over the top
repeaters		repeaters			astride	

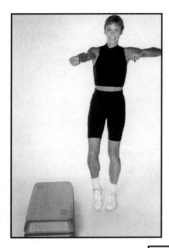

Figure 5.1 Tap down.

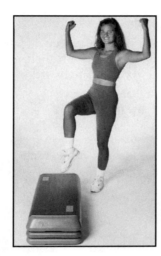

Figure 5.4 Chest press (vary arms).

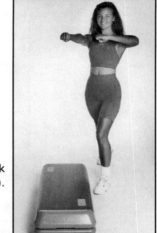

Figure 5.2 Lunge back (vary legs).

You should start simple, gradually develop 4- and 8-count patterns, and piece them together. One advantage to this method is that it allows you to relax and anticipate what will happen next. The following are options for sequencing multiple-skill patterns.[5, 6]

Double-Skill Sequence (Two Step Patterns Combined)

Use two base skills to form a two-part step pattern.

Two-Part Step Pattern Combination.

Directional approach: from the side.

✣ **Turn step** (length of bench) (see Figures 4.32–4.35).

✣ **Over the top** (width of bench) (see Figures 4.36–4.39).

Begin by performing four 8-count cycles of each move, and break it down from four to two to one 8-count cycle.

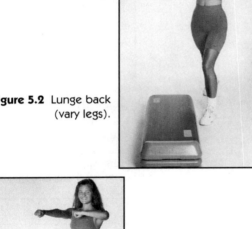

Figure 5.3 Knee up (vary legs).

Multiple-Skill Sequence

Use three or more base skills in a sequence. Examples of multiple-skill sequences with three-, four-, or five-part step pattern combinations are:

Three-Part Step Pattern Combination.

Directional approach: from the front.

∻ Base step (Figure 5.5)

L	R	L	R	
Up	up	down	tap down	alternate

∻ Bypass knee front (Figure 5.6)

L	R	R	L	
Up	**knee up**	down	down	alternate

∻ Diagonal travel knee front (Figure 5.7)

L	R	R	L	
Up	knee up	down ¼ turn	down	alternate

Four-Part Step Pattern Combination.

The three-part step pattern combination described can become a four-part step pattern by adding:

∻ Diagonal knee repeaters (Figures 5.8 and 5.9)

L	R	R	R	R
Up	**knee up**	**tap down**	knee up	tap down

R	R
knee up	down & turn

NOTE: When following the combinations diagrammed on an empty bench, the numbers that are circled ⓞ are non-weight bearing steps, and the numbers that are double-circled ⓪ and labeled indicate bypass moves.

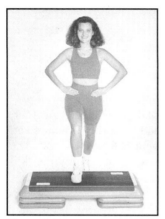

Figure 5.5

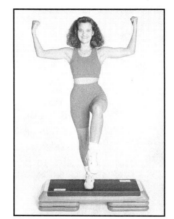

Figure 5.6

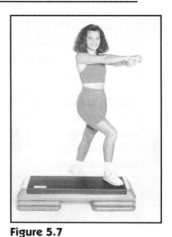

Figure 5.7

Three-Part Step Pattern Combination depicting a base step, bypass knee front, and diagonal travel knee front.

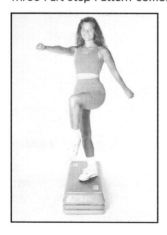

Figure 5.8

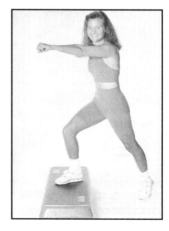

Figure 5.9

Four-Part Step Pattern Combination depicting the knee up and tap down of diagonal knee repeaters.

Five-Part Step Pattern Combination.

Directional approach: from the side.

Figure 5.10 illustrates an empty bench with sequential placement location of each foot. Beginning at the bench's end with your right side to the bench, weight on the **left** foot on the floor, step on the bench to the #1 location with your **right** foot.

✦ Steps 1–4: **Inside end to outside end** (see Figures 4.48–4.51). Cue: "step up to middle, up, step down forward, tap down"

✦ Steps 5–8: **March backward on the floor.** Cue: "march back"

✦ Steps 9–12: **Single lead step with bench tap** (side approach). Cue: "step up, tap up, step down, tap down"

✦ Steps 13–16: **Turn step** (see Figures 4.32–4.35). Cue: "up, up 1/4 turn, down, tap"

✦ Steps 17–20: **Over the top** (see Figures 4.36–4.39). Cue: "up, over, down, tap"

NOTE: When repeating this pattern, you will be facing the opposite direction and you will begin with your weight on the right foot on the floor and step on the bench with your left foot.

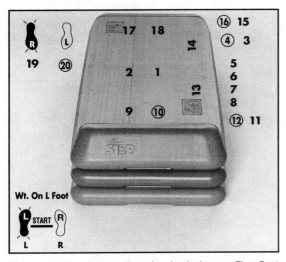

Figure 5.10 Empty Bench depicting a Five-Part Step Pattern Combination.

Five-Part Step Pattern Combination.

Directional approach: from the top.

Figure 5.11 illustrates an empty bench with sequential placement location of each foot. Begin by standing on top of the bench at the bench's end facing it.

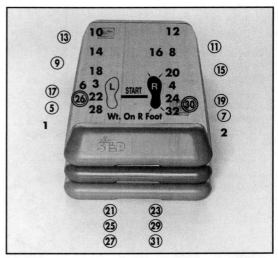

Figure 5.11 Empty Bench depicting a Five-Part Step Pattern Combination.

✦ Steps 1–4: **Straddle down** (see Figures 4.27 and 4.28). Cue: "out, out, in, in"

✦ Steps 5–12: **Lunge side move forward** (see Figure 4.29). Cue: "tap side, left and right, move forward"

✦ Steps 13–20: **Lunge side move backward.** Cue: "tap side, left and right, move backward"

✦ Steps 21–24: **Lunge back off the end** (see Figure 4.31). Cue: "tap back, left and right"

✦ Steps 25–32: **Double knee repeaters.** Cue: "tap back, knee up, left and right"

Advanced Step Choreography[7, 8]

Advanced step patterns utilize various bench orientations/approaches and can be challenging because of the changes in the lead leg and weight-bearing leg.

"Handlebar" Step. (Figures 5.12–5.15)

Directional approach: from the front.

L	R	R	L
Up	**tap up**	**down side**	down tap
L	R	R	L
Up	tap up	**down back**	**down**
			(step out wide to other side)

Repeat on other side.

Box Step. (Figure 5.16)

Directional approach: from the side

R	L	R	L
Outside leg up	up	down	down

NOTE: May progress to a single/ alternating base step to the front by performing a 1/4 turn when the outside leg steps up.

Step, Touch, Straddle to Other Side. (Figure 5.17)

Directional approach: from the side.

Figure 5.17 illustrates an empty bench with sequential placement location of each foot.

R	L	L	R
Up	tap up	step down	step down
(1)	(2)	(3)	other side (4)

L	R	R	L
step up	tap up	step down	tap down
(5)	(6)	(7)	(8)

Double "T" Step (Figure 5.18).

Directional approach: from the end.

All base steps and basic step patterns can be used to create an 8- or a 16-count step pattern that incorporates **all three sides** of the bench, begin-

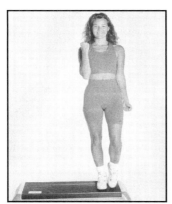

Figure 5.12.
R tap up

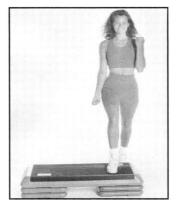

Figure 5.14.
R down back

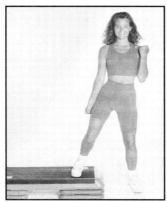

Figure 5.13.
R down side

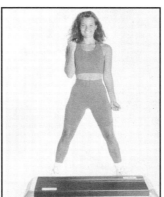

Figure 5.15.
L down

"Handlebar" step

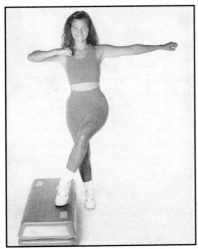

Figure 5.16. Outside leg up (step 1) of Box Step.

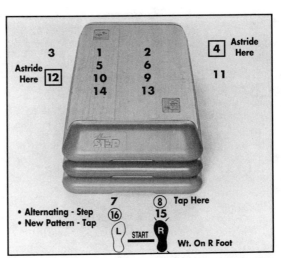

Figure 5.18. Empty bench depicting Double "T" step.

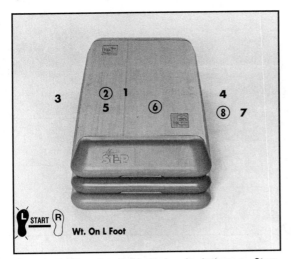

Figure 5.17. Empty bench depicting a Step, Touch, Straddle to Other Side step.

with the pattern, placing your next foot on top of the bench, or on the side or at the end on the floor, wherever the sequential number indicates foot placement.

NOTE: **When repeating the pattern, final step #16 takes weight onto L foot. The next move is Up (R).** *When changing to create a totally new pattern, final step #16 is a non-weight-bearing move (like a tap), with the next weight-bearing step on that same (tap) foot, either in place on the floor, or up, on the bench.*

---

ning from the end of the bench. When you get creative, your back should never face the bench while stepping up. Only three sides of the bench are available to you for any one pattern.

Figure 5.18 illustrates an empty bench with sequential placement location of each foot. Beginning from the bench's end and with your weight on your **right foot** on the floor, step up on bench to the #1 location with your **left foot**. Continue

❖ **SUMMARY**

The possibilities for step training combinations are endless. The base steps and basic step moves are simple, but combining the steps in various ways can be challenging. By adding variety, such as propulsions, traveling and repeater moves, and arm gesturing, you can vary the intensity to meet your fitness level. Create your own step patterns by using Chart 5.1, "Creating Your Own Step Training Pattern Variations."

⟡
CHART 5.1

Creating Your Own
Step Training Pattern Variations

Directions: Following all of the guidelines in Chapter 4 and 5, create your own patterns. For safety reasons, only three sides of the bench can be used in a pattern. Start with a bench approach from the end, front, side or top, and proceed incorporating multiple basic step patterns and multiple bench approaches.

⟡ Indicate the location of the weight-bearing foot (WBF) to start the pattern, freeing the other foot to then be step #1.

⟡ Begin the pattern by locating a "1" up on the bench (or down on the floor), followed by the location of the next step, identified as "2."

⟡ Continue locating steps 3–8, then 9–16, identifying any step that has a key directive (e.g., ⑧ is a tap non-weight-bearing move; [12] is an astride position).

⟡ Identify any bypass step movement with a double circle around the non-weight-bearing foot location and labeling the type of bypass move (e.g., ⑤ fwd. kick).

⟡ List arm gestures to accompany each step movement, plus any additional choreographed pointers (sounds, etc.) below, at right. Enjoy being creative!

STEPS:

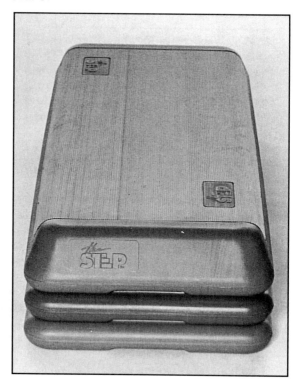

ARM GESTURES TO STEP #:

1. _____
2. _____
3. _____
4. _____
5. _____
6. _____
7. _____
8. _____
9. _____
10. _____
11. _____
12. _____
13. _____
14. _____
15. _____

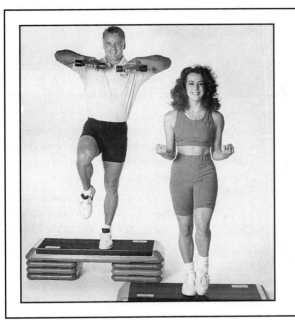

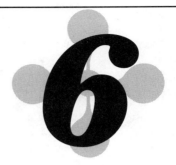

The Next Step: Variation

The underlying structure of an effective step training program has been established. It can be exciting now to build upon that basic success strategy by adding appropriate change or **variation** to your program. The following list identifies some of the key reasons you'll want to include variety:

- ❖ progressing from the status of beginner to intermediate, or intermediate to advanced, in both aerobic capacity and motor skill level;
- ❖ biomechanical needs (e.g., rehabilitation from injury);
- ❖ physiological needs (e.g., resuming after an illness);
- ❖ psychological needs (e.g., increasing the difficulty of a workout to keep you continually mentally and physically challenged).

❖ VARYING THE INTENSITY

Step training enables you to design a program that will continually improve your overall fitness, whether you are a beginning, an intermediate, or an advanced stepper, and all within the same setting. It is simply a matter of knowing *how to adjust the intensity* of what you are doing. (Intensity, again, is directly reflected by heart beats per minute, or rate of perceived exertion.)

As you continue to do the simple base steps, basic step patterns, and most of the step pattern variations, *intensity can be increased or decreased* to accommodate your individual needs (regarding fitness, skill, health status, or goals), by changing any of the following variables:

- ❖ raising or lowering the bench height;
- ❖ using or not using hand-held weights;
- ❖ using long- or short-levers;
- ❖ using high- or low-impact steps;
- ❖ using difficult or easy arm movement range-of-motion levels;
- ❖ increasing or decreasing the music tempo or beats per minute (not a variable the *individual* has control over in a group setting).

This chapter tells how to increase and decrease intensity applying these variables, for the beginning, intermediate, and advanced stepper. Beginners are regular exercisers who have never done step training, intermediates are regular step trainers, and advanced refers to skilled, regular step training participants.[1]

BEGINNING STEP TRAINERS

Before beginning a step training program, your fitness level must be determined as detailed in Chapter 1. Based on the results of the fitness assessment, you will have a better idea how quickly you can expect to progress by varying the intensity in your step training program.

As a beginner participating in step training for the first time, to ensure safety, select a 4" or 6" bench and concentrate on performing just the foot movements. Omit the arm patterns altogether by keeping your hands on your hips.[2]

Next glance down and watch the bench and your feet, as to where they are to move *next*. When you are comfortable with the step height and the step moves, you will be able to step safely and efficiently in the right location without constantly looking down at the bench.

If you become temporarily fatigued or cannot follow the step patterns, lower the platform or perform the moves just on the floor, until you recover your breath or timing and coordination.

INTERMEDIATE STEP TRAINERS

If you have regularly engaged in beginning step training and can now safely and efficiently use good form to complete a step session, consider any of the following to increase your intensity, or workload, to sustain the training zone heart rate:

∻ increase step height in 2" increments (see Chapter 2);

∻ increase music tempo gradually from 118 BPM to 125 BPM (see Chapter 2);

∻ intensify arm movements by using a larger range-of-motion (see next section);

∻ add light 1–4 pound hand-held weights, starting light and progressing slowly (presented later in this chapter);

∻ vary footwork (presented later in chapter).

These variables should be added only one at a time.

ADVANCED STEP TRAINERS

From research findings conducted by fitness professionals, product literature promoting the correct use of the equipment involved, and the professional experiences of both authors, the following are the *maximum safe limits* (to date) when step training:

∻ bench height: 12"

∻ hand-held weights: 4 pounds

∻ music tempo: 128 BPM

∻ step pattern variations that include high-impact (propulsion) moves: 8–16 counts of continuous repetitions, followed by low-impact steps for at least 4–8 counts, before resuming high-impact moves.

∻ High-range arm movements: 8 counts of continuous repetition, followed by at least 16 counts of middle- or low-range moves, before resuming high-range moves.

These maximum limits for the advanced step trainer are achieved steadily, over time and are progressively changed or added, one at a time.

INCREASING ARM MOVEMENT INTENSITY

All step training arm movements are similar to those used during strength training and always must be performed in a controlled manner. Intensity can be increased *significantly* by the type of arm movements.

The joint from which the arm movement originates determines the intensity. *Long-lever* arm movements originating from the shoulder provide more intensity than *short-lever* moves originating from the elbow.

The *range-of-motion* of the arm movements directly reflects the more and less intense moves.

Low-range moves (Figures 4.73–4.80), in which elbows remain near the waist and sides, are the least intense. *Middle-range* moves (Figures 4.81–4.92), in which the elbows are kept at chest level, provide more intensity. *Upper-range* arm movements (Figures 4.93–4.101), in which the elbows are shoulder high and above the head, provide the most intensity and increase in workload.

Because arm movements classified as upper-range tend to escalate the heart rate higher than the accompanying work reflects, the number of upper-range movements should be limited. Enough methods to escalate intensity to challenge your workload are available without continually doing upper-range arm movements.

ADDING HAND-HELD WEIGHTS TO INCREASE INTENSITY

Another means of adding intensity to stepping is to use light, 1–4 pound hand-held weights (Figure 6.1).[3] Adding hand-held weights not only increases intensity and improves cardiorespiratory fitness but also *increases upper body muscle tone and strength*. This is the reason step training is considered a *total body workout*. Training-effect benefits are achieved in all of the muscles of the body simultaneously.

Because step training is predominantly (and can be totally) low-impact and performed at a moderate tempo, hand-held weights can be incorporated safely by strictly following these safety precautions.[4]

1. Add hand-held weights of 1 or 2 pounds *only after* you are proficient at step training and when you have achieved an intermediate level of fitness and skill. The key criteria for using weights is that you must maintain *good body position the entire time*. When form declines, immediately omit using the weights.

2. Do not use hand weights if you:
   - ❖ have high blood pressure;
   - ❖ have a history of coronary disease;
   - ❖ have low pack pain;
   - ❖ have arthritis;
   - ❖ have other chronic or temporary orthopedic problems;
   - ❖ are past the first trimester of pregnancy;
   - ❖ are significantly overweight.

3. When you begin using light weights, use them for just one routine per session, and gradually build up your endurance. Start low and go slow.

4. Begin by using slow, small ranges-of-motion with short-lever, non-rotational arm movements, and never use flinging or uncontrolled movements.

5. Avoid maintaining arms at or above shoulder level for extended periods (i.e., overuse of tendons that stabilize the shoulder joint and unnecessary blood pressure elevation).

6. Avoid full-arm extension moves in short counts of music time.

7. Avoid using weights while performing propulsion steps.

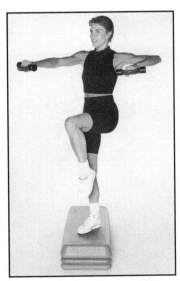

Figure 6.1. Adding hand-held weights to increase intensity.

8. Feel free to put down weights during your workout at any time. Place them safely under the bench or where you'll not accidentally step on them.

VARYING FOOTWORK

Another key way to modify exercise intensity is to vary specific footwork and impact. Lunge-steps, traveling movements, and repeaters create a higher intensity than other step patterns tested.[5, 6] All high-impact moves (when you are momentarily airborne and landing on one or two feet — e.g., propulsions) create a higher intensity compared to low-impact footwork, when at least one foot is always on the ground or bench.

APPLYING INTENSITY PRINCIPLES

The following figures illustrate how to vary (increase or decrease) the intensity of base moves and basic step patterns[7] by varying the arm and leg levers and range-of-motion used.

Changing Intensity Movement #1: Step Touch Bypass

Directional Approach: diagonal **4 count.**

Low (Figure 6.2)

    L   R   R   L
Up   **tap up**   down   tap down
(hip joint used in low range-of- motion)
Arms: Bicep curl (low-range, short-lever)

Moderate (Figure 6.3)

Change tap up to **knee up** (increased hip range-of-motion, short-lever leg); change arms to shoulder-high lateral raise (mid-range, long-lever arms).

High (Figure 6.4)

Change knee up to front **kick** (long-lever leg); change arms to forward and overhead, reverse "L" position (upper-range, long-lever arms).

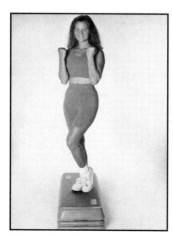

Figure 6.2. Low.

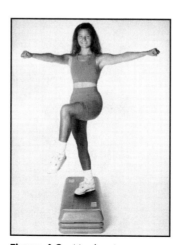

Figure 6.3. Moderate.

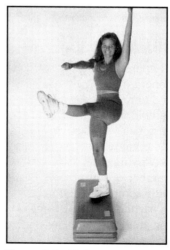

Figure 6.4. High.

Changing Intensity Movement #2: Side-Lunge
Directional Approach: from the top.

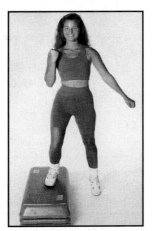

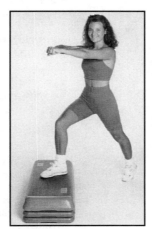

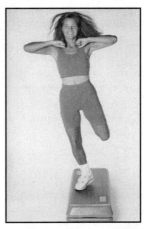

Figure 6.5. Low — Perform a **grounded lunge**. Body faces forward, foot parallel to bench; arms press down when you step down (low-impact).

Figure 6.6. Moderate — Perform a lunge with a small **hop** and ¼ turn. Opposite arm punches forward. Alternate sides and arms (high-impact).

Figure 6.7. High — Perform a lunge with a small **propulsion** (a lift with an airborne turn to land in a lunging position) (higher impact).

SUMMARY: VARYING INTENSITY

Appropriate exercise progression is a key component in adhering to exercise — sticking to it — and preventing exercise-related injuries. Your aerobic fitness level, skill level, health status, and personal needs or goals determine when you can incorporate variety.

Varying the step training workout offers a number of advantages. First, it allows participants with completely different fitness levels and needs to participate in the same class. Second, by providing many options to accomplish individual program needs, participants are motivated to work within their own fitness and skill levels. Finally, it allows everyone to immediately see improvement in cardiovascular endurance (the ability to perform more repetitions and work for longer periods), strength development of the musculoskeletal system, and performance improvement of the motor skills involved in step training.

This first option has shown you how to increase and decrease intensity, the amount of work you do, measured as heart beats per minute. To *increase* intensity, exercisers safely and progressively work toward ultimately using the maximums presented, unless physical limitations prohibit. To *decrease* intensity, the lesser or minimums in the variables are selected.

✛
STEP/BENCH WITH STRENGTH

Options for using the step/bench are unlimited. It can be used not only for aerobic conditioning (as has been presented) but also during the anaerobic phase of the workout for improving muscle strength and endurance through strength training (Figures 6.8 and 6.9). To complement the cardiovascular step portion of the workout, include progressive resistance training techniques *using the step/bench in conjunction with a variety of equipment* such as hand-held light weights, elastic tubing, and bands.

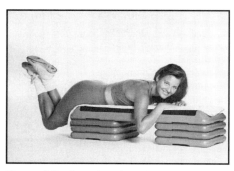

Figure 6.8. Step Bench with Strength.

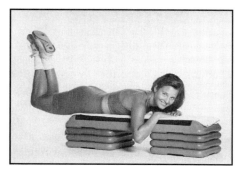

Figure 6.9. Step Bench with Strength.

BENEFITS OF STEP/BENCH WITH STRENGTH

Key benefits to be attained by adding a progressive resistance strength training program to the step aerobics workout are:[8]

✛ develop stronger muscles to help with the tasks of daily living;

✛ improve resiliency (elasticity);

✛ restore and maintain muscle balance (to prevent injuries);

✛ improve body composition (greater lean, less fat ratio);

✛ increase firmness and tonus of muscles (greater bulk and definition);

✛ overall well-being and functional efficiency (feel better and move easier).

When combined with other strength training equipment, the bench/step can be an innovative piece of exercise equipment. Three advantages in using it when performing strength training exercises are:[9]

✛ provides support for the pelvis, low back, and neck, which increases effectiveness and decreases the chance of injury;

✛ affords the opportunity to work with or against weight resistance by letting gravity work for or against you;

✛ increases the range-of-motion possible for each exercise, allowing greater muscular contraction. (Because of the elevation of the step, you can extend the movements and get a "prestretch" for full range-of-motion.)

THE PRESCRIPTION FOR STRENGTH TRAINING EXERCISES

The strength training segment is optional in the step aerobics class setting, but because it is a vital component of total physical fitness, most step aerobics classes today include 10–20 minutes of strength-training to provide a well-balanced and complete fitness program. Guidelines from the American College of Sports Medicine state: "Strength training of a moderate intensity, sufficient to develop and maintain fat-free weight, should be an integral part of an adult fitness program. One set of eight to twelve repetitions of eight to ten exercises that condition the major muscle groups, at least two days per week, is the recommended minimum."[10] Thus, the prescription for more fully developing your lean (fat-free) weight is:

Strength Training			
Set	Reps	Varieties of Exercises	Minimum Days/Week
1	8–12	8–10 targeting major muscle groups	2 (with max.: 4/week, or every other day)

The strength training segment in a step aerobics setting focuses on the following isolated muscle groups of the upper and middle body. (Because the lower body, which includes the hips and buttocks, thighs, and lower legs, is used extensively during step training, exercises to develop strength in the lower body are not presented in this text.)

⋅⊹⋅ Upper body: chest, upper back, shoulders, arms;

⋅⊹⋅ Mid section: abdominals, lower back;

Exercises presented here use the following types of weight resistance modes:

⋅⊹⋅ Commercial rubber resistance bands;

⋅⊹⋅ Commercial rubber resistance tubing alone, or with the aid of the bench;

⋅⊹⋅ Gravity-assisted techniques, in which the bench is placed in an incline or decline position, with 1–4 pound hand-held weights, resistance tubing, or using your own body weight as the sole resistance.

Note: The bench is not designed for using free-weights that weigh over ten pounds.[11] And, for comfort and safety, place a towel on the bench platform when lying on it.

The exercises illustrated and described here have been categorized according to the location of the muscle group(s) benefited (upper body/midsection) using a variety of equipment. Figure 6.10 illustrates the major muscle groups[12] to be strength-trained, and Table 6.1 on page 79 identifies the exercises that will accomplish the training.

VARIETY OF RESISTANCE

To incorporate variety into your program, try using all of the following forms of resistance:

1. *Your own body (or parts)* lifted and lowered[13] against gravity as the weight resistance, as in push-ups or curl-ups (see Figures 3.16 and 3.21). To progressively increase the resistance involved in lifting your body's weight against gravity, a strategically placed free-weight is used (i.e., on the sternum for a curl-up, Figure 6.32, or between the shoulder blades for a push-up, etc.).

2. *Hand-held weights* (not wrist-weights) are used in controlled movement or placed on the body in the key locations to add weight resistance to the body part being lifted and lowered.

3. *Rubber resistance bands,* 9", 12", or 16" long, in widths of ¼–1½ inches can be used. The length and width are selected according to whether the exercise is for upper or lower body, and for your current strength fitness level in the muscle group being trained.

4. *Rubber resistance tubing,* approximately 3–4½ feet long so you can adjust it according to your height in a range of light to heavy thickness that you select according to your current level of strength fitness.

Muscle Structure[12]

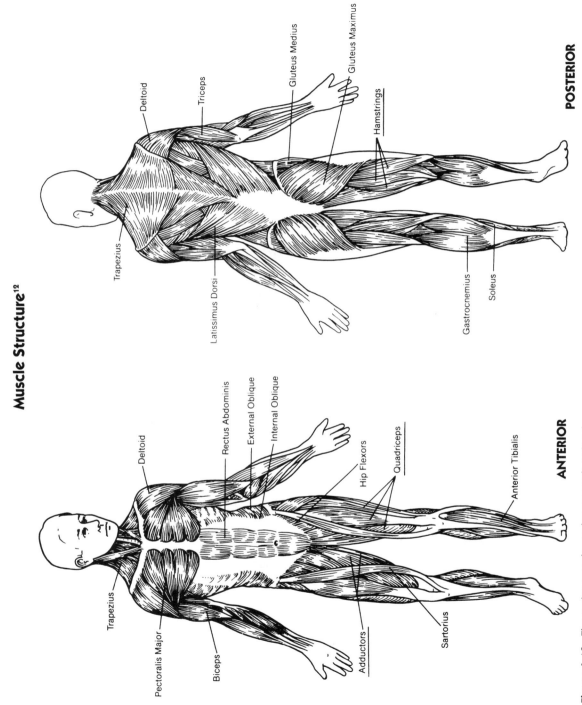

POSTERIOR

Deltoid

Triceps

Gluteus Medius

Gluteus Maximus

Hamstrings

Trapezius

Latissimus Dorsi

Gastrocnemius

Soleus

ANTERIOR

Deltoid

Rectus Abdominis

External Oblique

Internal Oblique

Hip Flexors

Quadriceps

Anterior Tibialis

Trapezius

Pectoralis Major

Biceps

Adductors

Sartorius

Figure 6.10. The major muscles to be strength-trained.

5. You also may *combine all the above*, using a step-bench in a level position, or in the gravity-assisted incline or decline positions. You will begin to realize from the exercises shown that the possibilities for variety in the strength training segment are fun, exciting, inexpensive, and unlimited.

Options 3, 4, and 5 are shown in Figure 6.11. Following are the principles for using these unique pieces of equipment.

Using Resistance Bands and Tubing

The general directions for using either resistance bands or tubing are:

✦ Select bands and tubing based on your fitness level.

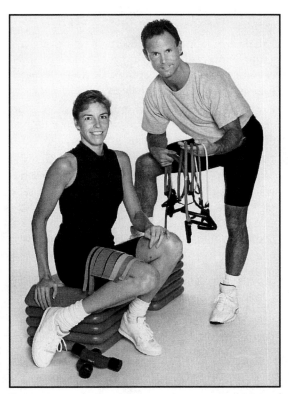

Figure 6.11. Various equipment to use for resistance when exercising.

✦ Always inspect the bands and tubing before each use for nicks and tears that may arise from continued use.

✦ Never, under any circumstances, tie pieces of band and tubing together.

✦ Always exhibit proper body alignment and posture while exercising.

✦ To assure safety, keep your face turned slightly away from the direction of movement.

✦ While performing single-limb upper-body movements, always anchor the band between one hand and the thigh, hip, side, or shoulder, depending on the movement.

✦ Always anchor the tubing under the ball of one foot or both feet (when not using it with the bench), depending on your level of fitness and the desired amount of tension you wish to create.

✦ Always control the bands and tubing, especially during the return phase of the movement. Do not let them control you.

✦ Perform 8–10 repetitions of each exercise. When using one arm or leg, switch sides so the same muscle group is worked an equal number of repetitions on the opposite side of the body. Be sure to work all muscle groups with equal intensity and repetitions at each session, to avoid muscular imbalance.[14]

Bands

Bands (Figure 6.12) are available in a variety of sizes to vary the intensity of your workout.[15] Suggested sizes:

✦ Beginner
⅜" upper body (pink or light blue)
⅜" or ⅝" lower body

✦ Intermediate
⅝" upper body (light blue)
⅝" lower body

✦ Advanced
¾" upper body (dark blue)
¾" lower body

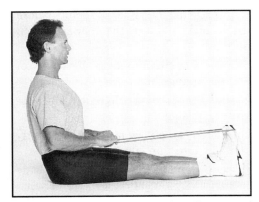

Figure 6.12. Seated lower leg flexor and extensor — using a rubber resistance band.

Tubing

Tubing also is available in a variety of sizes to vary the intensity of your workout.[16] Suggested sizes:

⊹ Beginner
  Very light and light tubing (yellow or green)

⊹ Intermediate
  Light and medium tubing (green or red)

⊹ Advanced
  Heavy tubing (blue)

PRINCIPLES OF STRENGTH TRAINING

If possible, plan approximately 10–20 minutes for strength training during your workout, applying the following principles:

⊹ Precede and follow muscle strengthening exercises by stretching exercises specific to the muscles that are made to work against resistance. Any muscle group strengthened by exercise also should be stretched regularly to prevent abnormal contraction of resting length.[17]

⊹ Of key importance, stabilize your joints and your spine before beginning each exercise.

⊹ Perform each movement using a smooth, continuous, full range-of-motion action for the joint/muscle group involved, and keep the timing of the movement (usually slow) totally under your control. Ballistic (rapid or jerky) movements increase the risk of injury.

⊹ For proper timing take approximately 2 seconds to perform the overcoming-resistance-action (concentric) phase, and from 2 to 4 seconds (i.e., at least the same time, or up to twice as long) during the release or lowering (eccentric) phase to return to the starting position of each exercise.[18]

⊹ Exhale during the lifting, overcoming resistance-action move; inhale during the release or lowering and return. (Exception: During overhead pressing movements, inhale as you lift).[19]

⊹ Use visualization and self-talk here. Plan your concentrated thoughts to accompany your lifting/exhale and lowering/inhale movements.

⊹ Design the repetitions of each exercise and the sets of repetitions according to the progressive resistance format. Begin with one to three sets of 8–12 repetitions for most exercises. (Exception: For abdominal work, begin your program by performing two sets of 15–30 repetitions per set). Select 8–10 exercises that condition the major muscle groups of your body for at least two of your aerobic sessions per week, if you have no other separate strength training program.

⊹ When you become jerky, are not smooth, continuous, and rhythmical in the move, and are not using the full range-of-motion possible around your joints, you've completed your lower limit possible for that set. Make a record of this number. This lower limit becomes the baseline to which you attempt to add more repetitions as soon as possible.

❖ It will later be less beneficial if just more repetitions are performed without adding additional resistance. Adding resistance in increasingly greater increments (i.e., from 1–4 pounds if using hand weights, or thicker rubber if using bands/tubing) will provide the added resistance you need over the course of your program. In the step aerobics class setting, however, don't go over the 4-pound limit for hand-held weights if this is your choice of resistance equipment.

❖ Perform strength training on isolated muscle groups on an every-other-day basis. Your muscles need a day to recover, so don't incorporate a program to strength train with resistance (weights/bands/tubing) daily. An alternative to this program is to perform strength training exercises with resistance (weights/bands/tubing) for the upper half of your body one day, and for the lower half of your body the next day. You thus are alternating the days the muscles are strength training.

❖ Allow brief rest periods between bouts of vigorous exercises. This is the most efficient way to improve strength. (The time-frame for rest is defined as regaining a normal breathing pattern.)

TIPS FOR INCLINE AND DECLINE POSITION EXERCISES[20]

❖ Be sure bench blocks are locked into place.

❖ Make sure there is no more than two blocks' difference from one end to other.

❖ Place a mat or towel on top of the bench platform.

❖ To sit on the bench, place your pelvis in the middle of the bench platform, then adjust your hips.

❖ Use your hands to push your torso up when in the decline position.

❖ Avoid the decline position for prolonged periods of time.

❖ Maintain tension in the tubing by securing it under key parts of the bench and wrapping extra tubing length in your palm.

TABLE 6.1. Strength Training Exercises Using Various Forms of Resistance with Step/Bench

UPPER BODY Chest/Upper Back/Shoulders/Arms (Figures 6.13–6.31)	MID-SECTION Abdominals/Low Back (Figures 6.32–6.34)
Chest Press Bent-Arm Chest Cross-Over Chest Fly Straight-Arm Side-Raise Overhead Press Overhead Triceps Extension Deltoid Raise with Bent Knees Upright Row with Bent Knees Triceps Kick (Press) Back with Bent Knees Biceps Curl with Bent Knees	Gravity-Assisted Curl-Up with Weights Reverse Curl-Up Back Extension

---

Chest Press (Figures 6.13–6.14)
BENCH AND TUBING (Pectoralis Major, Anterior Deltoid, Triceps)

NOTE: This is an excellent beginning exercise to develop pectoral strength.

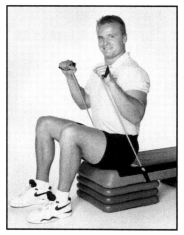

Figure 6.13

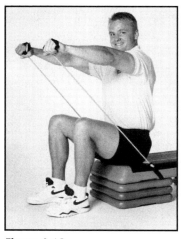

Figure 6.14

Position: Loop tubing under the step/bench so an end is accessible on both sides. Sit facing outward on the end of the step. Grab a handle in each hand, taking up slack by wrapping the tubing around your hands. Bring your hands shoulder-high, elbows near sides.

Action: Exhale and press away, shoulder-high, straight out in front of you. Inhale and return.

NOTE: The step/bench is adjustable. For all strength training exercises using an incline / decline bench (four block risers at one end, two block risers at the other end), you'll get a fuller range-of-motion as you go through each exercise, allowing greater muscular contraction.

Bent-Arm Chest Cross-Over
(Figures 6.15–6.16)
INCLINE BENCH AND TUBING (Pectorals)
Adjust bench so two blocks are at low end and four blocks are at high end.

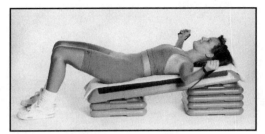

Figure 6.15

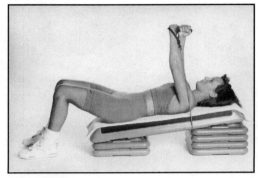

Figure 6.16

Position: Sit center; move buttocks to lower third of bench; lie with head resting at top. Grasp the tubing that is placed under platform center, near shoulders. Place your feet flat on the floor, with knees in open position, with arms wide open at shoulder level, elbows bent.

Action: Cross-punch arm position over chest while pressing your back firmly against bench. "Big-hug" position.

Chest Fly (Figures 6.17–6.18)
INCLINE BENCH AND 1–4 LB. HAND-HELD WEIGHTS (Pectorals)

Position: Lie on back with buttocks on low end of bench, knees in open position. Hold one hand weight in each hand above the shoulders, with the arms slightly bent, and wide open.

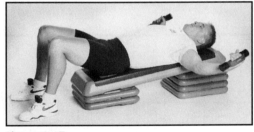

Figure 6.17

Action: Raise weights toward each other directly above you.

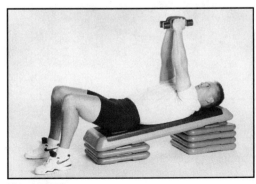

Figure 6.18

Straight-Arm Side Raise
(Figures 6.19–6.20)

INCLINE BENCH AND TUBING (Deltoids)

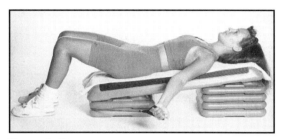

Figure 6.19

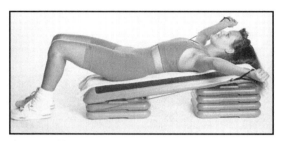

Figure 6.20

Position: Place tubing in the top notch, between platform and first block, at the low end of bench, giving a little tug to be sure it is secure. Roll up tubing, holding onto the handles, thumbs facing in toward bench.

Action: Gently lift up until the thumbs face up and above the head. Hold. Lower back to floor.

Overhead Press (Figures 6.21–6.22)

INCLINE BENCH AND TUBING (Deltoids/Triceps)

Position: Prone, with tubing in back of first block's

Action: Press up and forward, ending with thumbs rotating in, and facing each other.

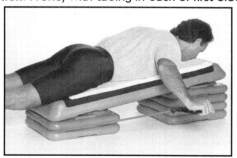

Figure 6.21

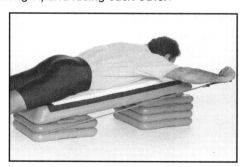

Figure 6.22

groove, hands starting at sides, wide, and chin resting on incline bench top.

Overhead Triceps Extension

(Figures 6.23–6.24)

INCLINE BENCH AND TUBING (Triceps)

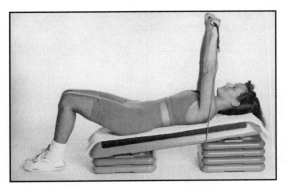

Figure 6.23

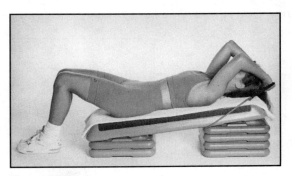

Figure 6.24

Position: Place tubing under center of bench so it is next to top blocks and at shoulder height. Raise arms so elbows are in the air and actually pinch in toward each other. The thumbs will start facing the ground.

Action: Extend up and rotate the palms up toward the ceiling. Thumbs will come up so they face each other. Relax back down. Cue yourself: "Up, press, contract."

NOTE: Bent knees in all of these illustrations assist in keeping a target heart rate, so these exercises can also serve as one-minute strength training "intervals" in an aerobic step training with strength intervals program. Interval training is presented later in the chapter.

Deltoid Raise with Bent Knees

(Figure 6.25)

BENCH AND TUBING (Deltoids/Trapezius)

Position: Stand on top of bench feet slightly apart with tubing under center, having fists top/thumbs-in-and-down position.

Action: Press up, bending knees, with elbows bent and hands leading, going only to shoulder level or lower. If fatigued, raise arms just half way, or use lighter tubing.

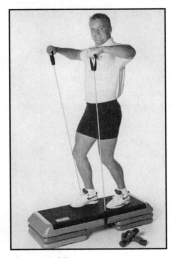

Figure 6.25

Upright Row (Figures 6.26–6.27)
BENCH AND TUBING (Deltoids/Trapezius)

Position: Stand on bench's center/back, feet together, with tubing under center, hands/fists now facing thighs.

Action: Raise handles up to chin, flaring elbows out slightly shoulder high, keeping spine firmly erect. Bend knees on action.

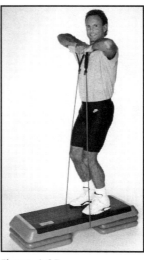

Figure 6.26   **Figure 6.27**

Triceps Kick (Press) Back with Bent Knees
(Figures 6.28–6.29)

BENCH AND TUBING (Triceps)

Position: Stand on the back third of bench with tubing under center/back. Palms start at sides on thighs, thumbs up.

Action: Rotate palms out and back to extension, thumbs down. Bend knees on the action.

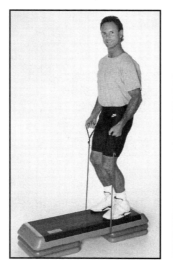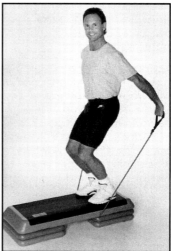

Figure 6.28   **Figure 6.29**

Biceps Curl with Bent Knees
(Figures 6.30–6.31)

BENCH AND TUBING (Biceps/Brachialis)

Position: Stand on the back third of bench with tubing under center/back. Hand/fist position now facing thighs.

Action: Curl up to sky, rotating palms on the way up so they face shoulders. Reverse the rotation for return. Again, bend knees on the action to increase heart rate.

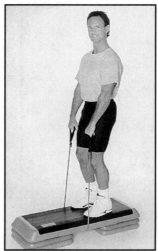

Figure 6.30   Figure 6.31

Gravity-Assisted Curl-Up (Figure 6.32)

INCLINE BENCH AND 1–4 LB. WEIGHTS
(Abdominals)

Position: With bench in incline position, straddle and sit on the lower third. Place 1–4 pound free-weights* on sternum (breastbone), with knees flared out wide and heels together, flat on floor. (This leg position works the abdominals and decreases the chance that the hip flexors will help in the movement.)

Action: Keeping lower back on bench at all times, curl-up, head looking forward. Hold, and contract with your mind thinking ("squ-e-e-e-ze"). This is all the farther you go; release and curl back down to lying position.

   *Adding more weight resistance is optional, but if you do, this is where it should be done. When using weights while on bench, maximum weight is 10 pounds.

NOTE: Repetitions for abdominal work can be 15–30, and two sets — one before a step aerobics session and one after, because the type of muscle tissue located here responds well to more repetitions for "definition" than other groups of the body. These exercises are to help strengthen sensitive lower back; the low back is completely supported during the abdominal contraction. No "daylight" shows between the bench mat (or towel) on the bench and your shirt in low-back area.

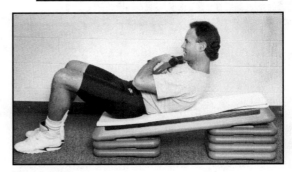

Figure 6.32

Reverse Curl-Up (Figure 6.33)
DECLINE BENCH (Abdominals)

Position: Place bench in a decline position. Lie on bench, face up with head at lower end of bench. Grasp lip of platform and top block over your head. Legs are skyward, with hips, knees, and ankles softly bent.

Action: Contract abdominals and raise buttocks, keeping lower back on the platform. Lower. Remember to breathe evenly during all strength training exercises. To hold your breath and turn red is never acceptable, as your working muscles constantly need oxygen.

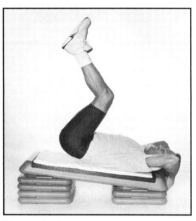

Figure 6.33

Back Extension (Figure 6.34)
INCLINE BENCH (Erector Spinae)

Position: Lie prone, with hips on lower third, legs extending off bench, supported by toes on floor. With chin on bench, place hands at hips area.

Action: Contract low back and raise upper chest. Hands may move in a sliding motion backward. Lower.

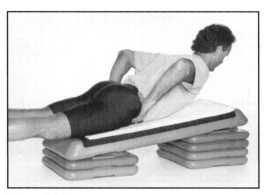

Figure 6.34

SUMMARY: STEP/BENCH WITH STRENGTH TRAINING

A second means of adding variation to your step aerobics program is to include a segment on strength training to fully develop the strength and endurance of skeletal muscles. More than a dozen exercises primarily targeting isolated muscle groups in the upper and middle body were given, all of which can involve using a variety of resistance equipment with the step/bench. Exercise prescription for strength training established by the ACSM, was the basis for the principals and guidelines presented.

Begin strength training slowly, methodically, and in absolute control of the amount of resistance or weights you are using. You will progress by using increasingly more resistance. You should record the exercises you perform, plus the number of sets, repetitions, and the type and amount of resistance used with each exercise. (Many of the exercises are shown with tubing, but the exercises also can be done using resistance bands or 1–4 pound hand-weights.) Charting your progress will give you a visual blueprint for success and a means of continual motivation.

Strength-fitness training to more fully develop muscle strength and endurance is a long-term project[21] calling for a dedicated personal commitment of many hours, just as the programs of stretching for flexibility improvement and step training for aerobic capacity improvement are. All fitness programs are for life.

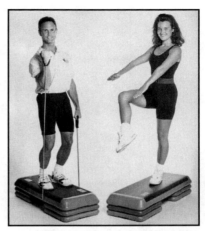

Figure 6.35. Step and strength interval training.

⊹ ━━━━━━━━━━━━━━

STEP AND STRENGTH INTERVALS

Step and Strength (Figure 6.35), a third program option, combines step aerobics with strength training using light resistance (tubing, resistance bands, or 1–4 pound hand-held weights), performed in a unique interval-training format. This option produces an excellent total fitness workout in a short time.

The interval training workout follows this format: *3 minutes of high-intensity step aerobics conditioning* (Figure 6.36), followed immediately by *1 minute of strength training* using the bench and resistance equipment described earlier (Figure 6.37). *These 3-minute/1-minute intervals are repeated at least five times in a complete high-intensity workout time of 20 minutes.* During the entire 20 minutes, your heart rate is kept in the training zone.

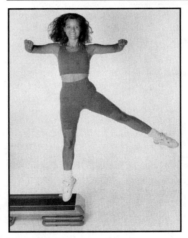

Figure 6.36.

Step

and

strength.

APPLYING INTERVAL STEP AND STRENGTH

Place the tubing (or resistance bands/hand-weights) under the step/bench. After your warm-up (see Chapter 3), do the first interval of step aerobics for 3 minutes (Figure 6.38). Then pick up the tubing and secure its position under the bench block's ends or under the center of the platform, whichever the exercise requires.

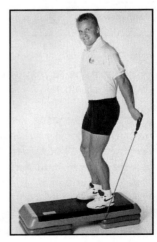

Figure 6.37.

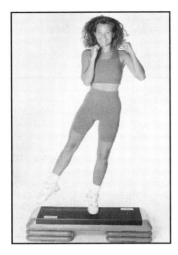

Figure 6.38. Step aerobic intervals — 3 minutes.

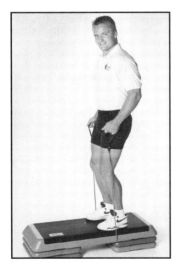

Figure 6.39. Strength training intervals — 1 minute.

Perform the strength move by first positioning your feet comfortably apart (Figure 6.39), either a bit astride or side-by-side. Then with an exhale, press, and hold while you maximally contract the muscles used. Every time you perform against resistance, use your mind as well as your body to achieve the full contraction. Telling yourself "up-sque-e-e-ze-and-*hold*" helps to attain the full contraction. Return to the original position with an inhale ("and-re-l-a-x"), breathing every time and continually.

While you press against resistance, maintain a little "squat," or *bending of the knees*, to keep the heart rate elevated and stay aerobic (continually using oxygen for your energy needs). To make sure you challenge yourself to perform to your maximum during every interval, take several "active recovery" heart rate checks during the 20 minutes. This will ensure that you are staying within your target heart rate zone at all times.

If you become fatigued during the strength interval, take a break or bring your arms up into position just half-way. Because step aerobics is lower-body intensive and these muscles get a big workout, *the strength interval focuses only on the muscles of the upper body*. After the strength interval, replace the tubing (bands, weights) safely back under the bench and perform the next step aerobics interval, continuing with this interval format for a minimum of 20 minutes.

Step and Strength is an extremely popular method of accomplishing a complete workout in one location in minimum time, using an easily planned program routine. It is especially helpful during times in your life when you don't have much time to fitness train.

⁜

TWO-STEP/BENCHES TRAINING

A fourth means of adding variety to your step training program is the advanced technique for experienced step exercisers only, who have developed a high level of skill (both form and technique), concentration, and endurance. This option, called "two-stepping" or "double-stepping,"[22] incorporates *two-step benches per person workout*.

Participants in two-stepping *use the center space between two benches* in addition to the outside floor space and tops of both benches to kick, prance, and tap up, down, over, and around the two benches. The suggested placement of the two benches is parallel to one another and 14" apart.[23]

No research to date has studied this new variation of stepping over a long term. Therefore, take *all of the precautions you normally do when trying an innovation.*

⊹
STEP AEROBIC CIRCUIT TRAINING

The fifth variation in your basic step training program consists of a *number of stations where specific exercise movements are performed in a predetermined time-frame of approximately 1–2 minutes.* When the station activity is completed, you immediately move on to the next station. The traveling time to the next station is also predetermined. When all of the stations have been visited in the allotted time, the circuit is finished. An advantage of this type of training is its versatility.

Step aerobics training circuits usually combine step training (to improve aerobic capacity) with weight training exercises (to develop muscular strength and endurance). By alternating the two modalities of exercise, the completed workout can yield the benefits of a total fitness regime.

How the circuit is planned is key to its success. A few guidelines are:

⊹ Alternate step aerobic stations with strength training stations.

⊹ Arrange stations so no two consecutive stations exclusively work the same muscle groups.

⊹ Maintain an elevated heart rate by moving quickly between stations.

⊹ Perform strength training exercises within your training zone heart rate, using light weights, quick repetitions, and *excellent form.* The focus at the strength training stations is to develop muscular endurance through many repetitions rather than to develop power using heavy weights.

⊹ *Attempt as many of the suggested stepping movement/patterns/sequences or strength training repetitions of a specific exercise as you can in the predetermined time.*

⊹ To improve, vary the circuits by *increasing* the:

  ⊹ number of stations;

  ⊹ planned step movements/number of reps performed, by allotting more time or speeding up the pace;

  ⊹ number of times the circuit is repeated;

  ⊹ amount of weight resistance used at the strength training stations or adding heavier hand-held weights to the step training movements (using a maximum of 4-pound weights).

SUMMARY OF THE NEXT STEP: PROGRAM VARIETY

The possibilities for variety in a *step training plus* program are unlimited. Within the parameters of safety, you can introduce variety to step training, using the exercise movements and equipment specified here as a take-off point.

The five possibilities presented were:

⊹ varying your *intensity*;

⊹ adding strength training through *weight resistance* variations;

⊹ *interval training* providing "step and strength" within the same routines;

⊹ *two-bench stepping,* incorporating two benches;

⊹ *circuit training* in which stations are set up to alternate step aerobic movements with strength training exercises, within a predetermined time-frame.

It is now time to tap into your own potential and consider what other possibilities exist for your program. Enjoy experiencing your unlimited creativity in action on page 90.

✛ Creative Program Additions ✛

✛

✛

✛

✛

✛

✛

✛

✛

✛

✛

✛

✛

✛

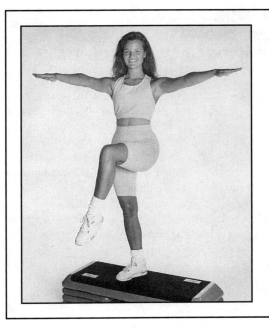

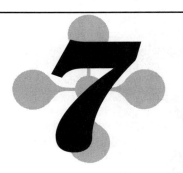

The Balancing Step: Healthy Choices

You have taken *a step in the right direction* by committing yourself to developing a fitness lifestyle, and experienced a *first step* toward fitness by understanding the principles behind the new exercise modality called step training. You've traveled *step-by-step* and learned many techniques, designed how and where to *step rhythmically to the beat*, and then taken the *next step* by adding significant variety to the step training basics. Your fitness journey is well underway!

Now is the time to take the *balancing step* incorporating all of these components with steps toward developing mental strategies to stay motivated, steps to keep your emotions in check through stress management and relaxation techniques, steps to ensure a balance between energy output and energy input through positive eating strategies, and steps to develop and maintain an ideal body composition through weight management techniques.

Achieving total fitness requires an understanding of the following components. Combined, they will enable you to make a complete range of healthy choices for a lifetime:

❖ The fitness mindset;

❖ Stress management and relaxation;

❖ Eating strategies;

❖ Weight management techniques.

❖ **THE FITNESS MINDSET**

*"To the possession of the self,
the way is inward,"* (Plotinus)

*We each must, therefore,
come of age by ourself.
Each must journey to find our
true center, alone.*

To develop a mindset for the fitness lifestyle, we first must become more aware of the choices we constantly make and what internal resources we use to make these choices. We, and others around

91

us, can experience directly the choices we make. We can clearly see, hear, and feel these responses. What we usually can't immediately detect is *how* — what process led us to those choices. Therefore, if we begin to consider the factors underlying our actions — the emotional forces, attitudes, beliefs, and programming already present and operating our "mental computers" — we can understand fitness for a lifetime and choose to incorporate it into our belief system or mindset.

First we must recognize the steps in the fascinating process we go through, in a split second, when we are faced with an immediate fitness choice in our daily lifestyle. ("Shall we take the stairs or ride the elevator up the two flights to the classroom today?") Taking the process apart, step by step, helps us to know where our mindset needs repair and allows us to change and insert new constructive possibilities. Let's begin this journey by taking a look at the self-management model[1] that identifies the underlying factors fueling and influencing our choices, and then establishing how to anchor a consistent fitness mindset.

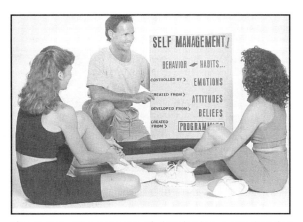

Figure 7.1. The process of developing a mindset for the fitness lifestyle includes becoming more aware of (1) the choices we constantly make, and (2) what internal resources we've used to make these choices.

BECOMING AWARE OF YOUR CHOICES: BEHAVIORS/ACTIONS/HABITS

Whatever we call it — behavior, actions, or habits — our choices are the end result of a unique problem-solving strategy we have within ourselves. A problem-solving strategy consists of how we perceive, store, and retrieve information about something. We initiate this problem-solving strategy by bringing the outside world inside us so we can interpret it. We do this by using our three predominant senses: visual (sight), auditory (hearing), and kinesthetic (bodily sensations, such as touch and muscle movements). To a much lesser degree we use our remaining two senses of taste and smell.

We blend these external sensory stimuli with the internal sensory stimuli stored inside of us. These internal resources include pictures or images (visual), self-talk (the auditory dialogue we constantly say to ourselves about what's going on), and emotions (kinesthetic, internal body sensations).

How you will problem-solve the fitness choices you make (or any choices you will ever make, for that matter) will come from your own internal thoughts: visual pictures you're making to yourself, auditory stimuli of external words and sounds or internal dialogue you're saying to yourself, and kinesthetic stimuli or body sensations you're experiencing or choosing to experience.

The lifestyle choices you make are, therefore, not made for you by someone or something else. *Your choices occur within you*, in that beautiful mental computer called your mind. "Because thought results in behavior immediately, the only control that is ever needed is thought control, and that entails only my present willingness."[2] The first step toward understanding how to make healthy fitness choices is becoming aware of all of the resources available for us to use, both externally and internally.

We must next filter out all the stimuli (both external and internal) that do not seem relevant at the moment to the problem at hand and focus only on what will fulfill our present, or most valued, wants or needs. (Again, this happens in fractions of seconds of time.) We complete this mindset process with a response: our *choice*.

We each, therefore, uniquely filter the multitude of sensory resources available to us and come up with "poor" or "healthy" choices. Clarifying what directly precedes our poor or healthy choices is the next step in this looking-inward process.

THE EMOTIONAL FORCES THAT DIRECT AND CONTROL OUR CHOICES

We each have an innate survival mechanism within us that strongly encourages us to avoid pain and gain pleasure.

Problem-solving anything in our lives usually consists of trying to remove the problem (pain) as quickly as possible so feeling good (pleasure) can again be ours. We often are not willing to endure the emotional pain that all self-discipline, growth, and change seems to require. We might say to ourselves, "Do I really have to do all these abdominal

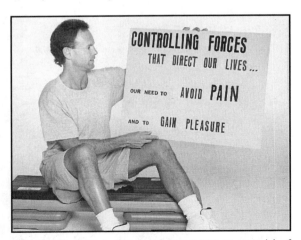

Figure 7.2. Pain is the force we want to get rid of quickly so we can experience the joy of feeling good.

crunches every day (pain of waiting for the gratifying results) to have a tight, toned abdomen, or is there a shortcut (to the pleasure of having the results)? I hate strength training (pain, either emotional or physical). Maybe if I just don't eat as many sweets, my abdomen will get smaller and look toned (instant pleasure gratification)."

A key to making and continuing a fitness commitment is to learn to accept delayed gratification (immediately having the results you desire long-range) and develop the growth and discipline (enduring the pain — delaying of immediate gratification) required for change — permanent, blueprinted change — to occur.

What creates the willingness to endure waiting for growth and change to happen?

YOUR ATTITUDE

The third step involved in the self-management development process entails examining our attitude. Your attitude — that perspective or lens of positive and negative, open and closed-mindedness, or enabling and disabling dispositions you take — is the true reflection of the opinion you have about something.

Choosing to establish or keep an open, positive mindset as a lifestyle is made possible by becoming keenly aware of your attitude toward problems and challenges you experience in everyday living. One of the ways you can do this is to listen and monitor — by writing down — your *self-talk*. Self-talk represents many ways to speak *to* yourself, out loud and silently within; and *about* yourself to others, out loud and in written and taped form.

We talk to ourselves 100 percent of our waking hours, about everything we're experiencing — seeing, hearing, emotionally feeling, and physically touching, tasting, and smelling. Negative self-talk is said or recorded using past and future tense verbs. Positive self-talk is stated and recorded in the present tense, using verbs ending in *ing*, creating the feeling that the present action is happening now.

In addition to self-talk, a second clear indicator of your attitude is experienced through your kinesthetic sense — *your physiologies and how you move*. For example, "When exercising . . . if you work hard and you're short of breath and keep saying to yourself how tired you are or how far you've run, you will indulge in panting or sitting down, which supports that communication. If, however, even though you're out of breath, you consciously stand upright and direct your breathing into a normal rate, you will recover in a matter of moments.[3]"

A third indicator of your attitude involves the *mental images or pictures you make*, how close/far away, color/black-and-white, moving/still, they are, and whether you are in the images (associated) or removed from the images and are observing (disassociated).

> Studies in neuroscience and psychobiology have shown that the way you think can affect your body and its performance. For example, stressful events perceived as threatening produce hormones in the body that reduce exercise efficiency and increase fatigue. However, when a stressful situation is viewed [pictured, imaged] in a more positive light, as a challenge rather than a threat, other chemicals . . . are released in the body, producing improved exercise performance.[4]

Once you're aware of how powerfully the factors that make up your attitude affect your adherence to a fitness program, you can do something constructive to improve them and thus bring about the changes you desire. It will be motivating to develop repetitive, positive self-talk (called *affirmations*), enabling physiologies (more effective postures and breathing techniques), and positive images (which are more colorful, close up, and active) that you are now choosing to hear, feel, and see about yourself and your program. If you are consistently delivering congruent messages to your nervous system that say you *can* do something, they signal your brain to produce the result you desire, and that opens up the possibility for it.[5]

The key thought with attitudes is openness — saying, picturing, and feeling "I can" and then remaining open for the answer to *how*. Your brain will continually search for possibilities when the channels and pathways are kept open. But just *telling* yourself positive affirmation statements, or *visualizing* helpful images, or engaging in various *motivational* movements regarding goals you would like to achieve (and actually *achieving* the goals) can be two separate phenomena — if your search for solutions stops there. It doesn't.

It's time to go one step deeper within and take a look at *what lies at the foundation of the entire mindset process*. What seed lies at the core of our choices?

YOUR BELIEFS: THE KEY TO UNDERSTANDING YOUR PROGRAMMING

Whether you call them guiding principles, rules for living, faith, philosophies for life, or truths you value, your beliefs ultimately determine the behavioral choices you make. What are beliefs?

⁺⁚⁺ statements that we have accepted as the truth and are useful, given to us by all the significant people in our life whom we trust;

⁺⁚⁺ commanders of the brain, which deliver a direct command to our nervous system;

⁺⁚⁺ the compass and maps that guide us toward our goals.

What is remarkable is that we continually make choices based on the programmed beliefs we have and value, and many times these beliefs are old, worn out hand-me-downs that we have accepted and never really questioned for personal validity. There is no universal rule stating that old, worn out, programmed beliefs can't be changed. Life *is* change and growth and involves stretching one's self to the limits of one's own potential.

People who have significantly changed history are those who have greatly changed our beliefs. Your beliefs can really help you change an unwanted behavior, especially if you have some key

new beliefs that work, are useful, and do not infringe upon the wants and needs of others.

Begin now to establish a collection of beliefs you have about living a healthy lifestyle. Stating, picturing, and feeling yourself believing these thoughts will assist you in blueprinting the fitness-for-life mindset.

❖ "This moment is a fresh, new opportunity. The past does not equal the future." (Tony Robbins)

❖ "The only definition for 'failure' is when I stop trying something altogether. I've reprogrammed all other ideas of failure (when I don't get what I wanted or needed) to mean I've just received 'feedback'/'results'."

Immediately preceding or underlying our choices, then, are our emotions, attitudes, and beliefs. This last resource we have stored within, our beliefs, constitute our ultimate valued guidelines for living that we have fully accepted and allowed to become programmed onto our own "mental tapes." *If we are to change our choices, we ultimately must update our disabling, no longer useful beliefs.*

The change process does not have to take a long time. Begin to more closely observe people who are successful role models of excellence and who exemplify the fitness lifestyle you would like to have. By duplicating their positive strategies, you will gain a shortcut toward achieving your own mindset for fitness. You will soon begin to realize that all healthy lifestyle choices or strategies are like time-honored recipes. They contain key ingredients, in defined measurable amounts, used in a prescribed order for consistently good results.

ANCHORING A FITNESS MINDSET

When you begin to consistently feel strong positive feelings by incorporating positive emotions, attitudes, and beliefs to make the choice for a healthy lifestyle, you will have a solidly programmed link, securely anchored into your thinking process. This blueprinting occurs first electrically, and then later chemically, onto your "mental map."

Reinforcing this link, or anchor, through repetition will more permanently solidify your newly blueprinted choice. You can achieve this by actually physically repeating the fitness choice, or through mental training — rehearsing the choice through audiotapes, imaging, and other means. *Change is a choice!*

New Beginnings

By doing what needs to be done right now,
we make the most of each present moment.
As long as we are alive,
we are always free to begin again.
Instead of following an old, worn-out habit,
make a fresh start this moment
on the rest of your life.
Each day is a new start.
Each moment is a beginning.

(Anonymous)

❖

STRESS MANAGEMENT PRINCIPLES AND RELAXATION TECHNIQUES

To understand potential and unlimited possibilities, we each must begin by setting a *standard* — establishing a starting point or basis — from which to grow. Your stress in balance or a balanced state of well-being expresses this ideal condition.

ESTABLISHING THE FOUNDATION

All of our world and universe is based on balance. Personal wellness is your life in balance. It requires actions, emotions, attitudes, beliefs, your will, and your power-source, all kept in mind and utilized in solving problems. Life balance or *wellness* is illustrated in Figure 7.3 as six components or balls that we need to keep juggling in the air, all at once. These six components are: physical, emotional, social, spiritual, intellectual, and talent expression. Each of these six components is an equally important contributor to the total balancing act we must engage in every day.

When any wellness component being juggled and kept in balance gets overlooked temporarily, or forgotten totally, it falls out of this balanced alignment and drops out of sight. We are then out of sync with life or get the feeling of not being whole. We've allowed one component or several components of our lives to take over and receive all of our attention. We soon experience the results: a decline in physical fitness, loss of a well-rounded social network of friends, or a boring, one-dimensional focus in our daily conversations.

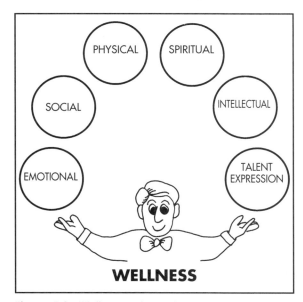

Figure 7.3. Wellness achieved through balancing six key dimensions of your life.

SUCCESS

How do we know if and when we are truly balancing all of these six areas of our lives? Developing a working definition for *success* — knowing when you've achieved this balance — is one way.

> *Success is the ongoing process of striving and growing to become more, in each of the dimensions of wellness, while positively contributing to others' needs.*

You can unconditionally believe that you are successful in anything you attempt in life if you (a) attempt and grow from it; (b) make more distinctions about what you're doing, and (c) accomplish it for the purpose of positively contributing what you've learned to others. By adopting this definition of success, it is difficult to feel like a loser or failure.

Consider the points mentioned. Life is an ongoing process, and wellness and success are landmarks in the journey. There is no one port or station in life, no one place to arrive at once and for all. The true joy of life is the trip. A port or station evokes a mental image to be held in expectation so we can tap into our unlimited potential for creative problem-solving. Life must be lived and enjoyed in the present moment as accomplished steps, as we go along. The final port will come along soon enough.

BALANCE IN BRIEF

The foundation of life is grounded in balance or a *wellness state*, composed of six dimensions: physical, emotional, social, spiritual, intellectual, and talent expression. Developing an all-encompassing definition for success in life affords us the opportunity to measure and know if and when we achieve individual life balance of the six wellness components. Developing this balance will satisfy our survival needs as well as our additional pleasure-filled wants.

What happens when we become imbalanced and stress enters our life? We must be realistic and aware that life will not be a continual, perfect balance, as life is not static and unchanging. Change is a constant. Thus, we must consider how to deal with imbalance when it enters our life.

STRESS: DEFINED AND MANAGED

Demands. Problems. Challenges. Change. Whatever you choose to call it, *imbalance* happens. Imbalance asserts itself daily and throughout our life, and we are left to react. *Stress* is our response. We cannot control the changes, demands, problems, or even the dirty deals we encounter, but we can learn how to manage certain situations so they are less offensive to us.

> *We can't control what happens to us, but we can learn to control our reactions to stress.*

Probably the most noted scientific researcher in modern times on the topic of stress and its effect on the human body is the late Viennese-born endocrinologist, Hans Selye. In his words: "Stress is the non-specific response of the body to any kind of demand that is made upon it."[6]

Good or bad, stress is our response to any kind of imbalancing that results from demands, problems, challenges, or changes. Therefore, scientifically and physiologically, stress is a *neutral* term. Positive stress, called *eustress*, is exemplified by running a marathon or seeing our loved one after many months at war. Negative stress, called *distress*, occurs, for example, when we experience a car accident or our home being vandalized. The goal in managing either kind of stress is the same as with all of life: to achieve a balanced state. This can be more easily understood using an analogy.

Stress management can be compared to playing a guitar. To play the guitar, we must use strings that come in a package, limp and with no tension on them (no demands or challenges). If there is no tension or stress on the strings, we can make no sounds. The same comparison applies to our lives.

If we have no stress, we have no challenges, no risks, no growth. Life is boring, and so are we, because not enough is going on in our life. But stretch those strings to their potential by placing them on the instrument with just the right amount of tension on them, add the human touch, and we will make beautiful sounds — harmony. Place too much tension on the strings (too many commitments on our time), and even the slightest pressure will cause the strings to pop — and so will we.[7]

To experience life with continual growth, it must have imbalance to create room for new possibilities. If we approach change from a positive perspective, it can open the doors to unlimited growth. If we take the negative view and see change as a threat to our comfortable stability, it can result in stagnation and imprison us in the depths of despair. The choice of perspective, and our subsequent reaction, is ours to make.

COPING SKILLS

How have you chosen to use your resources to cope (regain balance) when life has dealt you an imbalancing experience? Have you begun to realize that to stay mentally balanced, we all do *something* to cope with the stress in our lives? Your success in adjusting to and managing your response to stress can inspire growth and increased confidence to meet your next challenge (life situation). We each learn how to adjust to everyday small and big problems and life situations by using our vast internal resources. *We are not born adjusted; we systematically learn our adjustments.*

STRESS/TIME/LIFE MANAGEMENT

You can learn many effective strategies to manage stress. Developing your ability to relax is among the most important. Here is a guided imagery technique to following the positive stress of your workout hour, or to relieve the negative stresses you encounter every day.

⁘
GUIDED IMAGERY USING TOTAL BODY SCANNING

This technique utilizes your powers of control through your imagination. Your mind seeks out and recognizes tension and eliminates it through your ability to imagine the relaxation. It requires no physical exertion or planned tensing of muscle groups. Total body scanning has four steps: establishing the position; establishing the breathing pattern; tuning in to various parts of the body; and heart rate monitoring followed by simple static stretching to make you alert again (unless you use the technique before you go to sleep).

STEP 1: RELAXATION POSITION

⁘ Lie on your back. Figure 7.4. (You can also lie on the bench if your body fits; using the floor is easier, however.) If you feel uncomfortable because your entire back is not in contact with the floor, raise one knee up with your foot flat on the floor approximately 1 foot from your

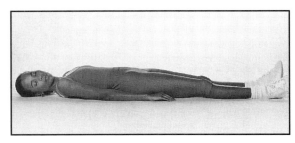

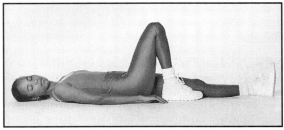

Figure 7.4. Relaxation position (option 1) lie on your back; (option 2) raise one knee to relieve the arched-back feeling.

buttocks. This knee-up position will relieve the arched lower-back feeling, especially for those with substantial buttocks or shoulder mass.

⁘ Turn your head slightly to one side. When you become totally relaxed, your tongue will relax backward and cover your windpipe if you keep your head straight in line with the rest of you.

⁘ Place your arms on the floor at your sides, palms down, with elbows slightly bent. Flexed joints are more relaxed.

⁘ Place your legs apart (not crossed or in contact with one another). As the legs relax, your feet will tend to roll outward.

⁘ If you relax best with your eyes open, keep them open. If you relax best with your eyes closed, close them. If you keep them open, focus continuously on one object only.

STEP 2: DEEP BREATHING

⁘ Take a deep breath and hold it in your lungs. Focus on the stretched-tight feeling you get in your chest by holding in the oxygen.

⁘ Now, slowly and purposefully breathe out (through puckered lips), a long, steady exhale. Create an image in your mind to lengthen the exhale. For example, see yourself blowing the fuzzy seeds off of a dandelion that has gone to seed or blowing a long, steady note on the flute.

⁘ Repeat this inhale, holding it, and follow with another slow, steady, long exhale. During this inhalation and exhalation, recognize that these next few minutes belong only to you. Do not share them with anybody or anything. Whatever problems, worries, or cares you have, including whatever you are going to do next in your day, briefly think what they are and list them all on a mental chalkboard in your mind. Then, mentally take out a big chalk eraser and wipe each of them off, one at a time, so you are looking at a blank chalkboard in your mind. Verbalize a thought to yourself (e.g., "This is my time now and you [problem] are just going to have to wait.") Then forget it during your relaxation technique.

⁘ Now follow your breathing cycle, whether it is fast, slow, regular, or irregular. Mentally tune in and follow each inhale and each exhale. Picture yourself in an elevator in which each exhale is a ride down one more floor (each inhale is the brief pause for the floor stop, door opening, and closing). Or imagine that your mind is on a slow roller coaster ride up and down, up and down.

⁘ Don't interfere with your inhalation and exhalation. As you begin to relax, the exhalation (breathing out) naturally becomes longer and longer. Ride with it and experience the longer ride out. This begins true relaxation.

⁘ At various times during the entire body scanning relaxation technique, mentally tune back in to your breathing technique, for mastering this "elevator ride" is essential to your relaxation.

STEP 3: TUNING IN

⁘ Start at the top of your head, travel down to the tips of your toes, and return to your midsection.

⁘ On the top of your head, mentally feel the "part" of your hair. Make it wide by relaxing your scalp.

⁘ Mentally envision your ears. Drop all tension to your ears. If you are wearing earrings, mentally feel them.

⁘ Tune in to your forehead. Is it tense and full of wrinkles? Make it flat and wide with no wrinkles. Picture it smooth.

⁘ What is the space between your eyebrows doing? Is it grooved and full of wrinkles? Relax. Make a wide space between your eyebrows. This is one of the telltale locations of human stress. A person who is highly stressed seems to permanently tense the space between the eyebrows (contracted, wrinkled). Calm, serene people stand out because this small space is wide, relaxed, and untensed.

⁘ Relax your eyebrows as if heavy weights were pulling down the ends. This also will relax your temple area.

⁘ A hinge joint near your ear hole opens and closes your lower jaw. Relax that mandible joint. It will make your jaw drop and your lips part. Relax your chin.

⁘ When you relax your jaw, mentally feel your teeth and tongue. When some people try to practice total relaxation, they tightly press (tense) their tongue to the roof of their mouths. Also, many people grit or grind their teeth at night, an audible sign of tension in the area.

⁘ Relax your throat by thinking of the feeling you get with the second stage of swallowing. People who sing or play wind instruments have been trained in this technique to relax the area, so realize that the best sounds will come out of a relaxed vocal mechanism.

⁘ Drop your shoulders and chest to make a wide space between your ears and shoulders. We unconsciously tense this area throughout the day. Whether we drive a car or walk in miserable weather, we tense the shoulders up near our ears, encouraging neckaches and headaches. When you think about it next time, untense these muscles if you don't actually need to hold them tensely.

⁘ Allow the weight of your chest to sink through to the floor. Think: heavy chest.

⁘ Drop all tension from your upper arms, elbows, lower arms, and hands until you can just feel your fingertips pulsating on the floor. You may feel a tingling in your fingertips.

⁘ Relax your buttocks. This is the key to untensing the lower half of your body.

⁘ Relax your kneecaps. This joint connects your upper and lower leg, and many times we tense the knee area when we attempt to relax other body parts. When you relax the knees, the upper legs will relax and the heavy weight of your legs will begin to drop to the floor. Likewise, the lower legs respond almost automatically, with the feet rolling outward.

⁜ Mentally feel what your toes are doing. Are they tensed and curled under? If so, stretch them out and then relax them.

⁜ Now return to the most difficult place to relax — the stomach and intestinal area. Direct your mind to the navel area and picture a wide, flat, picturesque pond. Envision a small pebble being tossed into the very center, creating a soft, rippling effect in which each ripple is a wave of relaxation. Feel the weight of your navel area sinking through, past your spine, onto the floor below you.

⁜ Return to your breathing cycle, and follow it several times. Focus totally on the long, slow exhale.

⁜ Rest a few moments and enjoy the totally untensed feeling.

STEP 4: HEART RATE MONITORING AND STRETCH

⁜ In this lying-down position, feel for your pulse. Mentally picture and feel your heart beating. Actively try to slow it down with your mind. Cue it to beat slower.

⁜ Count your pulse for 15 seconds and multiply by 4 for a minute heart rate count. How does this compare with your resting heart rate count after 6–8 hours of sleep? What does 3 minutes of relaxation do for your body's recovery from exercise or daily stress?

⁜ Before you get up, sit up slowly and stretch your arms, legs, chest, and back, so you become alert immediately. You must do this 15-second stretch or you'll find yourself yawning for an hour afterward. Of course, if you do this before going to bed, omit the stretch.

SUMMARY

Life is a journey of many steps. We desire the pleasure that balance gives us. We attempt to find ways to manage when imbalance (stress) enters the scene. A most enjoyable means of regaining the balance we seek is through relaxation techniques. Total body scanning, a technique of guided imagery, develops an awareness of our own personalized resources we have stored within to manage the stress of our lives.

The blueprint for mastery has been drawn. Practice is what will permanently program the management of your stress.

EATING STRATEGIES

"Choose what is best; habit will soon render it agreeable and easy." Ancient philosopher Pythagoras stated this principle of making choices, and it hasn't really changed today. Better or best choices are available for you to make. Let's look at the source of the energy used for your physical fitness workout, the energy you intake.

Your body has two basic types of nutrient needs:

⁜ Foods that satisfy your energy needs.

⁜ Foods that meet the needs for growth, repair, and regulation of body processes.

Nutrients are chemical substances that your body absorbs from food during digestion. Your body needs at least forty nutrients. *Diet* here means total intake of food and drink. *Essential* nutrients are those your body cannot make or is unable to make in adequate amounts. These must be obtained from what you eat and drink. If your diet does not properly provide them, your body cannot perform well mentally or physically.

This is where choice comes in. You may know what the better choices of foods are (called *nutrient-dense* foods[8]), but if you don't eat the best choices available, you really don't know good nutrition at all. Good health, optimum fitness, and good nutrition result from not just knowing what is best but choosing it 80 to 90 percent of the time.[9]

✣ BEST CHOICES FOR A BALANCED DIET

A well-balanced diet is one that contains the following six basic nutrients. Proper amounts of each are established according to your age, gender, activity level, and state of wellness:

✣ Carbohydrates

✣ Fats

✣ Proteins

✣ Vitamins

✣ Minerals

✣ Water

These nutrients can be supplied from one of two eating plans presented here: (a) *Food Guide Pyramid, A Guide to Daily Food Choices*, established by the U. S. Department of Agriculture,[10] and shown in Figure 7.5, or (b) the four food groups as illustrated in the pamphlet *Guide to Good Eating*, published by the National Dairy Council,[11] and shown in Figures 7.6–7.9. *The eating plan described throughout this chapter follows the guidelines presented in the latter plan.*

You cannot always take in all of the essential nutrients every 24 hours. What *is* important is that over a span of several days and weeks, you continually select from the four groups to meet nutrient needs.

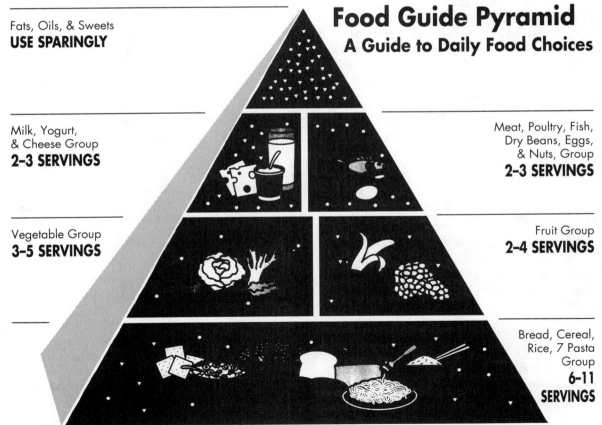

Food Guide Pyramid
A Guide to Daily Food Choices

Fats, Oils, & Sweets
USE SPARINGLY

Milk, Yogurt, & Cheese Group
2-3 SERVINGS

Meat, Poultry, Fish, Dry Beans, Eggs, & Nuts, Group
2-3 SERVINGS

Vegetable Group
3-5 SERVINGS

Fruit Group
2-4 SERVINGS

Bread, Cereal, Rice, 7 Pasta Group
6-11 SERVINGS

From U. S. Department of Agriculture

Figure 7.5. Food Guide Pyramid, A Guide to Daily Food Choices.

NUTRIENT DENSITY

Following the figures of each food group shown here, foods have been listed according to *nutrient density, the amount of nutrition per calorie each food provides*. To get the most nutrition for the least calories, choose foods from the four-star groups.[12] The categories are:[13]

4 stars = most nutrition per calorie

3 stars = next to most nutrition per calorie

2 stars = next to least nutrition per calorie

1 star = least nutrition per calorie.

If you know little about human physiology (how your vital processes work), it's best not to resort to chance or whatever nutritional guidelines you encounter. An abundance of scientifically-based, easy-to-read literature has been researched with controls and explains what balancing the needed basic nutrients entails. Select guidelines developed by well-established medical and fitness professionals rather than those from your favorite movie and television stars or supermarket trade magazines.

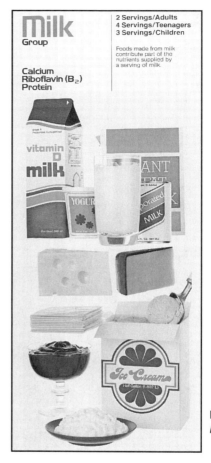

Figure 7.6.
Milk group.

MILK GROUP

The only group in which the serving sizes change in reference to your age is the milk group. Adults need two servings except: pregnant or lactating women need four servings; growing, pre-adolescent children need three servings; and teenagers need four servings. Calcium, riboflavin (vitamin B$_2$), and protein are the key nutrients needed to build the basic structure and strength of bones and teeth, assist in the production of energy needs, and help in the growth and maintenance of every living cell. If you are not an avid milk fan, you can eat any of the foods in the milk group and they will supply the calcium, riboflavin, and protein you need.

Rating:	Food Choices in Ranked Order:	Serving:
****	nonfat plain yogurt,	
	nonfat milk,	1 cup (8 oz.)
	lowfat cheese,	1 ounce
	buttermilk, lowfat plain	
	yogurt, 1%-2% milk	1 cup (8 oz.)
***	regular fat cheese,	
	ricotta cheese,	1 ounce
	whole milk, kefir, lowfat	
	yogurt w/fruit,	1 cup
	lowfat chocolate milk,	
	nonfat frozen yogurt	1 cup
**	pudding, custard	1 cup
	lowfat frozen yogurt,	
	ice milk	1½ cups
*	cottage cheese	2 cups
	milkshake	1½ cups
	Kissle	1 cup
	ice cream	1½ cups

Note: Nutrient density figured for **calcium**

MEAT GROUP

Even though this group is called the "meat group," plant foods eaten in combination can supply the needed protein, niacin, iron, and thiamine and represent an alternative to eating meat.

Some of the plant foods that can be combined so their proteins complement each other (allow the amino acids to combine to form balanced protein) are: dried beans and whole wheat, dried beans and corn or rice, peanuts and wheat.[14]

Everyone needs two servings per day of the meat group (except pregnant women, who need three servings per day). One serving is equal to 2 ounces of cooked lean meat, fish, or poultry, or the protein equivalent. Visually, a 2-ounce portion fills the palm of an average hand and is the width of the little finger.

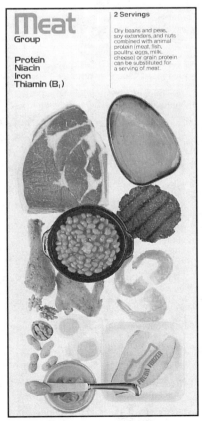

Figure 7.7. Meat group.

Cheeses are counted as servings of meat or milk, but not simultaneously. All excess fat should be removed from any meat you eat. You should remove the skin from poultry and eat only the meat, eliminating unnecessary calories.

Rating:	Food Choices in Ranked Order:	Serving:
****	lean cuts of: beef, veal, fish, pork, lamb, poultry (visible fat removed)	2-3 ounces, cooked
	eggs	2
***	regular and higher fat cuts of: beef, fish, pork, lamb, poultry, (visible fat **not** removed);	2-3 ounces cooked
	tofu	7 ounces
	dried beans, peas, lentils	1 cup cooked
**	nuts and seeds	½ cup
*	peanut butter	4 tbsp.
	hot dog, luncheon meats, sausage	2-3 ounces

Note: Nutrient density figured for **iron** and **protein**.

FRUIT AND VEGETABLE GROUP

This group provides vitamins A and C, which are actually catalysts or action starters. The most important functions are:

⁙ Forms and maintains skin and body linings.

⁙ Cements substances to promote strength in cells and hasten healing of injuries.

⁙ Functions in all visual processes.

⁙ Aids in the use of iron.

Everyone needs four servings per day. One serving is equivalent to:

⁙ Medium-size whole fruit or vegetable

⁙ 1 cup raw

⁙ 1/2 cup cooked

⁙ 1/2–3/4 cup juice

⁙ 1/4 cup dried fruit

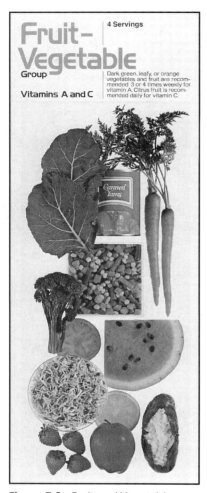

Figure 7.8. Fruit and Vegetable group.

Sources of Vitamin C

Fruits and vegetables such as broccoli, oranges, grapefruits, and strawberries are recommended daily for supplying the needed catalyst vitamin C. This vitamin is water-soluble, which means that if too much is taken in, the excess is excreted through the urine. If you decide to take vitamin C supplement pills in massive doses, your body reacts by increasing the level it needs. If you then suddenly stop taking vitamin C supplements, your body reacts as if it were deficient. Supplementation is costly and unnecessary for well people who eat properly.

Rating:	Food Choices in Ranked Order:
****	spinach, chard, broccoli, cantaloupe, tomatoes, brussels sprouts, asparagus, kale, green peppers, winter squash, romaine lettuce
***	vegetable juice, zucchini, green beans, oranges, cabbage, cauliflower, sweet potatoes, apricots, cucumbers, orange juice, carrots, grapefruit, celery
**	artichokes, strawberries, peas, corn, bananas, potatoes, beets, peaches, iceberg lettuce, sprouts, mushrooms, pears, avocados, pineapple juice
*	apples, raisins, grapes, canned fruit, dried fruit, french fries

Note: Nutrient density figured for **folic acid, vitamins A and C.**

Sources of Vitamin A

Orange and green. Two simple colors will help you remember that foods of these colors will provide vitamin A. Dark green, leafy, or orange vegetables and fruits (such as carrots, sweet potatoes, and greens) should be eaten at least every other day. Because vitamin A is stored in the fat tissue of the body, an overdose through supplementation in pill form can be fatal. (The same is true for the other fat-soluble vitamins, D, E, and K.)

GRAIN GROUP (WHOLE, FORTIFIED, ENRICHED)

Although this group assists with the growth and maintenance of cells and with the elimination process (fiber provides bulk to your waste for easy removal), the major function is to provide energy. Your number one daily need is energy to perform every daily function from sleeping to aerobics.

Four servings per day is the minimum amount required for everyone. If you do not use this carbohydrate food for the expenditure of energy, for growth and repair, or eliminate it, you wear it as body fat — future energy. It's like constantly carrying around extra gasoline for your car.

A minimum amount of four servings is suggested as a daily intake. A serving is not all you consume or serve yourself at one time but, rather, a measured amount of food. If you wish to lose fat weight, watch the amount of additional energy food you take in. If, however, you are an active person, such as a varsity or endurance athlete, you will want to provide an abundance of this energy food.

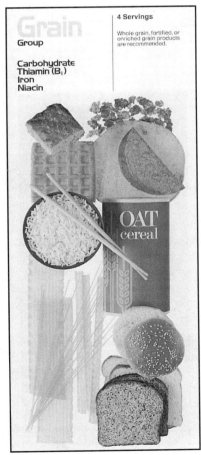

Figure 7.9.
Grain group.

Rating:	Food Choices in Ranked Order:	Serving:
****	bran (1/3 cup) and whole grain (1 cup) cereals,	1/3-1 cup ready-to-eat or 1/2 cup cooked;
	whole wheat breads and rolls,	1 slice or 1/2 bun;
	whole grain crackers,	4
	corn tortillas	1
***	pasta/noodles, brown rice,	1/2 cup
	enriched breads and rolls,	1 slice or 1/2 bun;
	cornbread	2" square
**	flour tortilla	1
	bagel	1/2
	plain muffin	1
	graham and saltine crackers	4
	pancakes	1
	other cereals	1 cup
	granola type cereal	1/3 cup
	pita bread	1/2 pocket
*	breadsticks (3), English muffin (1/2), enriched rice (1/2 cup cooked), biscuit (1), stuffing (1/2 cup cooked), croissant (1/2).	

Note: Nutrient density figured for **fiber**

COMBINATION FOODS

These items comprise more than one food group. They count as servings (or partial servings) of the groups from which they were made. Some of the food choices are: burritos, casseroles, chef salad, hamburgers, lasagna, macaroni and cheese, pizza, soup, stew, tacos. A new product line that presents an exciting choice is the vegetarian "gardenburger,"[15] to be listed under both the grain and protein food groups.

EXTRAS/OTHERS/ "SOMETIMES" FOODS

The foods classified as extras have no recommended number of servings. These food choices provide little nutrition and are often high in sugar, salt, fat, and calories. Classified as extras are: alcoholic beverages, bacon, bouillon, butter, cakes, candy, coffee, cookies, condiments, cream, cream cheese, doughnuts, fruit-flavored drinks, gelatin dessert, gravy, honey, jam, jelly, margarine, mayonnaise, non-dairy creamer, olives, onion rings, pickles, pies, popcorn, potato chips, pretzels, salad dressings, sauces, seasonings, sherbet, soft drinks, sour cream, sugar, tea, tortilla chips, vegetable oils.[16]

❖
MONITORING FOOD AND BEVERAGE INTAKE

Do you eat a wide variety of foods in moderation as shown in the Food Guide Pyramid or as described in detail from the "Super Four" food groups? Begin to formulate your eating plan. Start by thinking about what you had to eat today, and record the foods you ate in relation to the appropriate food group (can record on page 114).

For a combination food, think about what foods went into it, and list those foods under the appropriate food group. For example, the cheese on a pizza would be recorded in the milk group, the tomatoes and any other vegetables should be recorded in the fruit-vegetable group, and the crust is recorded in the grain group. The ingredients in a combination food may not always count as a full serving from the food group. Think in terms of quantity of servings, along with the nutrient category.

Continue monitoring your intake for one week. How does it measure up to the standards established for a balanced diet with special attention to selecting nutrient-dense foods? If your diet lacks variety, moderation, or foods from one of the food groups, you may not be getting all the nutrients and energy you need.

It's easy to improve your diet if you take it one step at a time. Start by choosing one challenge to work on, come up with a solution, and spend one week trying to correct it. After it's mastered, choose a second eating challenge that needs attention, and continue until you have a well-managed diet.

DIETARY GUIDELINES FOR AMERICANS

Food alone cannot make a person healthy, but good eating habits based on moderation and variety can help keep a person healthy and even improve health. The following guidelines suggested for most Americans, developed by the U. S. Department of Agriculture, Health and Human Services, are printed in more detail in the pamphlet, *Nutrition and Your Health: Dietary Guidelines for Americans.*[17] In brief, most Americans need to pay more attention to the following guidelines.

1. *Eat a variety of foods.* No single food supplies all the essential nutrients in the amounts you need. The greater the variety, the less likely you will be to develop either a deficiency or an excess of any single nutrient.

2. *Maintain healthy weight.* If you are too fat or too thin, your chances of developing health problems increase (e.g., high blood pressure, diabetes, heart disease, certain cancers). There is no one plan for maintaining healthy weight. If your concern is to lose fat weight, increase your physical activity, eat less fat and fatty foods, eat less sugar and sweets, and avoid too much alcohol.

3. *Choose a diet low in fat, saturated fat, and cholesterol.* If you have a high blood cholesterol level, you have a greater chance of incurring a heart attack. A population such as that of the United States, with diets high in saturated fats and cholesterol, tend to have high blood cholesterol levels.

   There is controversy about what recommendations are appropriate for healthy Americans. For the U. S. population as a whole, however, reducing our current intake of total fat, saturated fat, and cholesterol is sensible.

   ❖ Choose lean meats, fish, poultry, dried beans, and peas as your protein sources.

❖ Moderate your intake of eggs and organ meats (such as liver).

❖ Limit your intake of butter, cream, hydrogenated margarines, shortenings, coconut oil, and foods made from those products.

❖ Trim excess fat off meats.

❖ Broil, bake, and boil rather than fry.

❖ Read labels carefully to determine amounts and types of fat and cholesterol in foods.

❖ Consume 300 mg/day or less of cholesterol.

❖ Limit fat to 30 percent of daily calories or less. To determine the percentage of calories in a product that come from fat: 1 gram of fat equals 9 calories. Multiply the grams of fat in a serving times 9. The result equals the number of calories from fat in a serving. Divide the fat calories by the total calories in a serving to determine the percent. For example, if a chili label reads 1 cup serving = 200 calories/Fat 10 gm/Carbohydrate 5 gm/Sodium 980 mg.: There are 10 grams of fat in 1 cup of chili. 10 grams of fat × 9 calories = 90 calories from fat in 1 cup. 90 ÷ 200 = 45% of the calories in 1 cup of chili come from fat![18]

4. *Include plenty of vegetables, fruits, and grain products in your diet.* The major sources of energy in the average U. S. diet are carbohydrates and fats. Carbohydrates have an advantage over fats: They contain less than half the number of calories per ounce than fats.

Complex carbohydrate foods are better than simple carbohydrates. Simple carbohydrates (sugars) provide calories for energy but little else in the way of nutrients. Complex carbohydrates (beans, nuts, fruits, whole-grain breads) contain many essential nutrients plus calories for energy.

Increasing your consumption of certain complex carbohydrates also can increase dietary fiber, which tends to reduce the symptoms of chronic constipation, diverticulosis, and some types of irritable bowel. There is also concern that diets low in fiber content might increase the risk of developing cancer of the colon. Eating fruits, vegetables, and whole-grain breads and cereals will provide adequate fiber in the diet.

5. *Use sugars only in moderation.* The major hazard from eating too much sugar is tooth decay. The risk increases the more frequently you eat sugar and sweets, especially between meals, if you eat foods that stick to the teeth (sticky candy, dates), and if you consume soft drinks throughout the day.

❖ Use less of all sugars (white, brown, raw, honey, and syrups).

❖ Select fresh fruit or fruit canned without heavy syrup.

❖ Read food labels for sugar present: sucrose, glucose, maltose, dextrose, lactose, fructose, syrup. If it's listed as one of the first ingredients, it has a lot of sugar.

To determine how many teaspoons of sugar a product contains, 5 grams of sugar equal 1 teaspoon. Divide the grams in a serving by 5. For example, if a cereal box label reads 1-cup serving = 140 calories/carbohydrates/starch 10 gm/sucrose 15 gm/fiber 1 gm: There are 15 grams of sucrose in 1 cup of cereal. 15 grams of sucrose ÷ 5 = 3 teaspoons of simple sugar in 1 cup of cereal. Products are healthier when sucrose (simple sugar) amounts are low.[19]

6. *Consume salt and sodium in moderation.* The major hazard posed by excessive sodium is its effect on blood pressure. In populations where high sodium intake is common, high blood pressure is also common. In populations with low sodium intake, high blood pressure is rare. Establish preventive measures, such as:

❖ Eliminate all salt use at the table.

❖ Cook with little or no salt.

❖ Select foods that are low in sodium content.

The dietary goal for sodium intake is approximately 2,000–3,000 mg/day.

7. *If you drink alcohol, do so in moderation.* Alcoholic beverages tend to be high in calories and

low in other nutrients. Heavy drinkers may lose their appetite for foods that contain essential nutrients. Vitamin and mineral deficiencies occur commonly in heavy drinkers because of poor nutrient intake and because alcohol alters absorption and use of some essential nutrients.

One or two drinks daily seem to cause no harm in adults, but even moderate drinkers need to remember that alcohol is a high-calorie, low-nutrient food. If you wish to achieve or maintain ideal weight, alcohol intake must be well-monitored. Women should consume no more than one drink a day, and men no more than two drinks a day. Count as a drink:

❖ 12 ounces of regular beer

❖ 5 ounces of wine

❖ 1½ ounces of distilled spirits (80 proof).[20]

❖ ▬▬▬▬▬▬▬▬▬▬
SUMMARY

Diet is an essential facet of total fitness and wellness. Responsible eating plans are available from the sources named in this chapter. The axiom "the *application* of knowledge is power" applies here. Translating established guidelines and principles into practice will prove to be a powerful source of sustenance and energy that will enhance your physical fitness program.

❖ ▬▬▬▬▬▬▬▬▬▬
WEIGHT MANAGEMENT TECHNIQUES

We seem to readily admit that a primary goal in taking fitness courses is to *appear* healthy and slim. We desire this goal because we can directly see when our body looks nice, lean, and toned;

likewise, we can directly see when it looks out of shape and flabby. Many individuals therefore initially focus on a form of "fitness" or "being in shape" that they can readily see.

Your outer appearance, however, is not the entire, or even major, emphasis of a quality fitness program. You can live without well-toned muscles or a trim figure, but you can't live very long without a strong heart and lungs. Looking attractive and feeling good about your appearance are good ancillary goals. The key word, however, is *healthy* slimness. This requires developing a weight management program that you enjoy following, as the "final step" in achieving balance in your program.

 ▬▬▬▬▬▬▬▬▬▬
PRINCIPLES OF WEIGHT MANAGEMENT

Weight management means controlling the amount of body fat in relation to the amount of lean. Principles of weight management include: *weight maintenance* (keeping the same ratio of fat to amount of lean you're currently carrying); *weight gain* (almost always in terms of lean weight gain, not fat weight gain); and *weight loss* (always in terms of loss of body fat).

WEIGHT MAINTENANCE

In regard to weight maintenance:

❖ Your current composition of fat to lean is ideal for your best cardiorespiratory health.

❖ You are pleased with how you look. You have enough strength to function well in your daily life of work and recreation, to whatever extreme that may be. To remain at this constant weight, your energy must be in balance:

calories in = calories out

eating = expenditure; exercise

Because expenditure or "calories out" declines with aging (your metabolism slows down and you are less active), a decline in "calories in" (eating less) must accompany the aging processes.

WEIGHT GAIN

Weight gain almost always refers to gaining *lean* tissue, or thickening muscle fiber. When you want to look better cosmetically or to increase your strength for a sport or for daily needs, weight training is the type of activity in which to engage. If you are at an overfat weight, simultaneously *gaining lean weight and losing extra body fat will require you to eat less while increasing exercise* through weight training. Only if you are at ideal weight or underfat weight should you accompany this weight-gain program with an increase in caloric intake.[21]

Weight gain, then, means increasing muscle mass, or thickening muscle fibers. You do not gain more muscle cells; you thicken what you presently have.

WEIGHT LOSS

Weight loss refers to purposefully losing *fat weight*, never lean weight. Weight loss, of course, can be both lean and fat, according to how you go about losing the weight. Before you spend your money on any unique new weight reduction plan, claim, product, device, or book, call your local Better Business Bureau. If you completely understand the principles of weight loss, you will be able to determine a product's or program's worth before you spend time, money, and energy on it.

Principles of Weight Loss (Fat Loss)

1. *Fat weight is the only kind of weight to lose.* If a product or program claims to "get rid of excess body fluids," beware! Body fluids are not fat. Unnatural water retention, or edema, is a condition to be monitored and treated by a doctor, not by self-prescribed procedures or products.

2. *If water weight (fluid) is lost by sweating during exercise, it will and should return in 24 hours* to maintain the body's synchronized chemical balance. The energy-producing (metabolic) processes perform best when all of the necessary components are present. Dropping water weight is not effective weight loss. It is part of the fat-free weight and is vital to continuous well-being. You can understand, then, why weighing yourself after a strenuous exercise session is an inaccurate time to weigh.

3. *Fat is metabolized more readily and efficiently by performing moderate-intensity exercise for a long time.* If you are able to work continuously at a moderate intensity (lower end of your training zone) more than 30 minutes, you will tap into the most physiologically sound way to metabolize (burn off) that unwanted body fat. You need to exercise more than 30 minutes at a time to make significant changes in the fat content of the body.

   Wearing rubber suits, transparent plastic wrap around body parts, or heavy, long-sleeved sweats, nylons, or tights on hot days inhibits the free flow of sweat and does not allow it to perform its function of cooling. In hot and humid settings, wear as little as possible when performing fitness exercises. You cannot metabolize (burn up) fat faster by wearing more clothes.

4. *Fat burns off your body in a general way.* You can't "spot reduce." Spot reducing is perhaps the most prevalent misconception concerning fat weight loss. Many unscrupulous people defraud unsuspecting overfat Americans out of millions of dollars every year.

   By your genetic constitution, your body will use up its stored energy (fat) any way it is programmed to. You cannot do fifty leg lifts a day and hope to reduce the fat deposits in the area. You will shape up (thicken) the muscle fiber in the area, and toned muscles contain more of the enzymes involved in breaking down fat, but you do not burn off the fat there, or at any specific location. As energy is needed, it is withdrawn first from the immediate sources, and when this is used up, randomly from more permanent storage. It then is converted to an immediate usable form. Thus, at first you may lose weight in places you don't necessarily wish to, such as your face or chest/breast area. With perseverance, however, you'll burn off the fat in problem areas, too.

5. *Fat weight loss is accomplished most readily through a combined program of carefully monitoring your food intake and aerobically exercising.* When you monitor food intake (and eat less) and exercise (expend more calories or energy), you lose almost 100 percent fat. This is the only kind of weight you want to lose. Exercise speeds weight loss, not only by burning calories while you're working out but also by revitalizing your metabolism so you continue to burn calories more readily the next few hours.

It is difficult to lose fat weight by simply eating less food. If you do not exercise and severely restrict food intake only, the weight lost is not just fat. According to the way you have "dieted," your weight loss is approximately one-half to two-thirds fat loss and *one-third to one-half lean weight loss.* If your lifestyle and habits of eating and exercising don't change after you stop "dieting" and you gain back your lost weight, what you gain back is all fat. You are worse off because you lost both fat and lean and regained only fat. Over a lifetime of "yo-yo" crash dieting, the entire body composition changes to your detriment.

You can lose fat weight in many ways, but the only way to *keep* fat weight off is by having a regular exercise program.[22]

6. *Weight can be both gained and lost through an endurance exercise program.* You will burn off fat for energy and build up muscle simultaneously. Therefore, if you do not see a change on the scale immediately, don't be disappointed.

7. *A light exercise program tends to increase appetite, and a strenuous exercise program*

decreases appetite. After an endurance (aerobic) hour, the desire for food diminishes greatly. You will have time to carefully select or prepare what you know is good for you rather than ravenously grab that easy, high-calorie junk food sitting around.

8. *Eating less food is easier than exercising it off.* In most high-intensity fitness sessions, you will burn only about 300 calories. If you are seriously interested in losing extra fat weight, think twice about rewarding yourself with high-caloric treats afterward. Instead, replenish your water loss with noncaloric, yet quite filling, ice water.

9. *There is no such thing as a constipated endurance aerobic exerciser or athlete.* Regular, rhythmic stimulation of the entire digestion and elimination processes is one of the side benefits of step aerobics.

10. *The body's energy balance determines whether a person gains or loses body fat.* Proper weight loss is simply the result of taking in less caloric energy and expending more.

WEIGHT-LOSS STRATEGIES

A challenge such as being overweight may involve the need for (a) a better self-image, (b) a naturally slender eating strategy, (c) learning effective ways to become motivated and make decisions, (d) resolving a phobic response to childhood abuse, (e) learning better social skills, or (f) learning better coping skills.[23]

1 "NATURALLY SLENDER" EATING

One of the main differences between naturally slender people and overweight individuals is the construction of their mental images and self-talk concerning food. Overweight people usually construct present-tense pictures and self-talk. When they see, smell, hear, and experience food, they state internally, "Boy, am I hungry!" The result is that they immediately eat. They focus only on the pleasurable taste of food as they eat.

Naturally thin people usually do not have this present-tense strategy. They create future-tense pictures, self-talk, and feelings. They experience how they'll feel over time.[24] Those future pictures and words help them to master weight management, and they then can enjoy the pleasurable selections they do make.

2 CONTROL PANEL WITH ONE LARGE DIAL

The control panel was used in Chapter 1 to rate levels of perceived exertion. It can also be used to rate the level of relaxation or tension you feel at any one time. Or it can be used as an effective eating strategy, as shown here. Give each number a rating for how empty or full you feel before eating. Begin with the 5 representing "feeling very comfortable and full," and label in both directions from there. Here are some suggestions for labels, with a corresponding number to get you started, but you should label the control panel the way you want to, according to how you feel:

0-1	Starved/famished
2	The beginning of a meal
3	Only half-full
4	Not quite satisfied
5	**Feeling very comfortable and full**
6	Should have omitted extra helping, or dessert
7	Absolutely stuffed; ate and drank enough for two my size
8	Out of control temporarily
9	Out of control consistently
10	Body is plagued with chronic health risks from long-term overeating.

Then, when selecting and eating food, imagine your control panel and adjust it to how you feel currently, how you choose to feel during the eating process, and how you choose to feel when you're all done eating and drinking. (Figure 7.10)

CALORIC INPUT AND OUTPUT

Everything you eat or drink becomes "you" for either a short or a long time. You are what you eat. The food nutrients you eat maintain basic body functions such as breathing, blood circulation, normal body temperature, and growth and repair of all tissue. These are related to fixed factors such as age, body size, and physiological state. Any kind of caloric intake your body doesn't use or doesn't eliminate through solid or liquid waste is kept and worn as body fat for future energy needs.

CALORIC EXPENDITURE

Every moment of every day, no matter what activity you engage in, from sleeping to aerobically exercising, you are using up calories. Caloric energy expenditure is influenced most by how physically active you are all day. The body's basic needs are more or less fixed, but (the amount of) physical exertion is a personal decision.

How physically active your life is depends on your choices of profession and recreational activities. And most important, it depends upon a multitude of day-to-day choices: whether to walk to the local store or drive the car; use the stairs or elevator; rake the leaves or hire someone to do it; go out for a bicycle ride after supper or watch a TV show. How physically active your life is depends as much on attitude as it does on opportunity.[25]

FIGURING WEIGHT MAINTENANCE[26]

A. Record your present weight, in pounds.

B. Record your type of lifestyle; number values are:

12 = sedentary
15 = active physically
18 = pregnant/nursing
20 = varsity athlete or physical laborer

C. Multiply A times B:

This is your weight maintenance number, or the number of calories per day you need to eat to *stay* at your current weight.

CALORIC EXPENDITURES FOR VARIOUS ACTIVITIES

How many calories you burn per minute during any activity depends upon two criteria:

❖ *Intensity* (high-, medium-, or low-level work or exercise).

❖ *Body weight*.

The higher the intensity, the more calories you burn per minute. For example, you expend more energy and calories running a mile than you do walking that mile. The heavier you are, the more calories per minute you will burn (just as full-size cars burn more fuel per mile than small, compact models).

CALORIC INTAKE NEEDED TO GAIN LEAN WEIGHT

To add one pound of body muscle requires 2,500 calories. (This includes about 600 calories for the muscle and the extra energy needed for exercise to develop the muscle.) Thus, the daily caloric excess, over your maintenance number just figured, is 360.[27] You must be at or below your ideal weight to go on an excess calorie-eating program to gain muscle. You want to use your excess body fat first for your energy requirements.

To gain 1 pound of muscle:
2,500 calories equivalent to 1 pound of muscle
÷ 7 days in a week
= 360 daily excess calories to eat over maintenance intake number

---

Taking in more than 1,000 calories per day over the number needed to maintain weight, however, is likely to result in weight gain as body fat even if you are exercising strenuously on a regular basis.[28]

CALORIC INTAKE NEEDED TO LOSE BODY FAT

To lose more than two to three pounds of body fat per week is physiologically impossible.[29] Weight loss greater than this represents water and lean body tissue. To systematically drop unwanted extra body fat, you need to drop 3,500 calories a week, or 500 per day, to lose one pound of body fat per week.

To lose 1 pound of fat:
3,500 calories
÷ 7 days per week
= 500 calories a day less than your maintenance number

If you desire to drop more pounds per week but the total caloric intake would be less than 1,200, you need to re-establish your goal to lose only one pound per week. You never want to eat fewer than 1,200 calories per day. A daily diet of fewer than 1,200 calories is likely to be deficient in needed nutrients for you to grow, repair, stay well, and have energy to perform daily tasks and leisure activities. Sometimes, on a one-to-one basis, a doctor will have a patient eat fewer than 1,200 calories per day, but he or she will provide extensive guidelines and supplementation. This is *only* under the strict supervision of a doctor.

SUMMARY

To maintain a specific weight, caloric input must equal caloric output. To gain or lose weight requires an imbalance of energy in your eating and exercising lifestyle habits.

To provide a continual means of self-discipline concerning your weight control:

✢ Assess your weight whenever your lean or fat weight has increased or decreased substantially.

✢ Continue setting short- and long-range goals to achieve or maintain an ideal weight;

✢ Monitor your weight for changes, especially if you are prone to having difficulty in maintaining your weight.

Educating yourself about how to manage your weight can be interesting. It will help you understand how the human body works physiologically and how it doesn't work. You then can be alert to all of the false notions, especially of weight loss, that are rampant today. You can develop a program that will work for you for a lifetime!

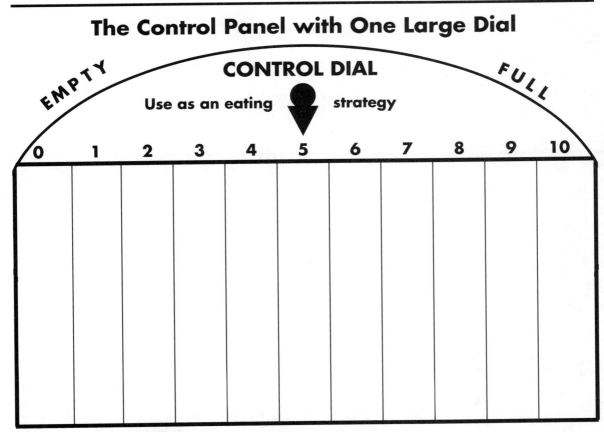

Figure 7.10. The Control Panel with one large dial.

MY DAILY CONSUMPTION

DATE/TODAY	/	/	/	/	/	/	/
MILK 1							
2							
MEAT 1							
2							
FRUIT & VEG. 1							
2							
3							
4							
GRAIN 1							
2							
3							
4							
TOTAL 1200 Calories From Above:	1200	1200	1200	1200	1200	1200	1200
Additional Servings Calories:							
Other ("sometimes food") Calories:							
TOTAL DAILY CALORIC INTAKE:							

(a)　What groups do you eat with consistent regularity? _____

(b)　Which groups do you tend to slight? _____

(c)　In which groups and categories do you tend to overeat? _____

(d)　Goal: _____

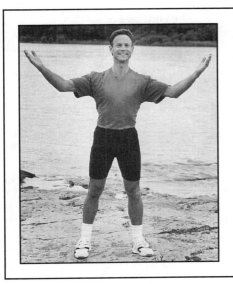

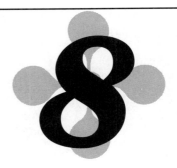

Future Steps: Goal-Setting

Your program is complete. You have learned physical fitness and mental training strategies on how to become fit and how to maintain that fitness. It's time to plan your future steps and challenge yourself by establishing your priorities and then setting your program goals. Knowing your priorities will help you to directly establish your goals — the pleasure-filled ends you are hoping to achieve in your fitness lifestyle.

 ## PRIORITIES

Priorities are the means to reach your goals. They refer to how you spend your time. Make a list of your top ten time priorities — how you *actually* spend your physical and mental energies each week. Rank-order them as to which priority is most-to-least important to you. Record any time-robbers that take you away from the priority. Can you identify a role model of excellence with whom you associate this priority?

Establishing Priorities

PRIORITIES are the means to your ends. They are things you give *time* to in the wellness areas of your physical/social/emotional/philosophical-spiritual/intellectual/talent expression dimensions.

-1- Top Ten Priorities (In Any Order)	-2- Hours Each Day	-3- Hours Each Week	-4- Time Robbers	-5- Rank Order of Importance	-6- Role Model
•				#	
•				#	
•				#	
•				#	
•				#	
•				#	
•				#	
•				#	
•				#	
•				#	

❖ GOAL-SETTING

Goal-setting requires you to ask yourself a few questions so you can set achievable goals.[1]

1. Ask yourself: "What will I see, hear, feel in regard to the results?" You'll recognize these as the components of motivation.

2. Ask yourself: "Why am I totally committed to achieving each goal?" Involve your values to answer this question. Values are any of the following: adventure and change, commitment, freedom, pleasure to others, happiness, health, love, power, prestige and worth, security, life purpose, success, talent expression, trust, loyalty.

3. Break the link of the old programmed ways by asking yourself: "What painful values do I choose to avoid?" Some of these pain-avoidance values are: anger or resentment, anxiety or worry, boredom, depression, embarrassment, frustration, guilt, humiliation, jealousy, feeling overwhelmed, physical pain, prejudice, rejection, sadness.

4. Re-establish the pleasure link by picturing, hearing, feeling: "Which actions do I choose to take or do immediately in each goal area, to master each goal? What is something I can start doing right now and within the next day?"[1]

This goal-setting procedure tells your brain precisely what goal you are choosing to set. It provides solid reasoning for why you're etching this goal-set groove. It also breaks old programming by presenting your pain-avoidance reasons. Last, positive action choices are made immediately to create the motivational pictures, self-talk, and movements necessary to initiate active change in your program. Making an audiotape for yourself by answering the goal questions for each goal you set may prove helpful. You'll find this "blueprinting process" to be a unique shortcut to achieving your goals!

Write your responses:

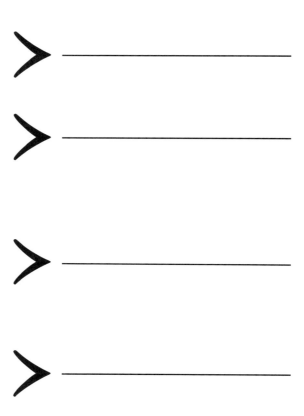

During this goal-setting process, one end to always keep in mind is to have *fun* during your pursuit of fitness excellence.

❖ SUMMARY

When they are properly internally set and continually nourished, goals will become reality. Believe it and you will see it. Your future resides within you as a rich resource of possibilities.

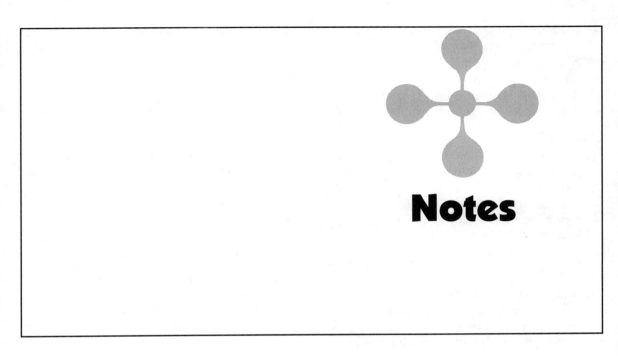

Notes

Chapter 1

1. Ralph Paffenbarger et al. *New England Journal of Medicine*, 314 (10) (March 6, 1986).
2. Kenneth H. Cooper, *Running Without Fear* (New York: M. Evans and Co., 1985), p. 195.
3. Kenneth H. Cooper, *Run Dick, Run Jane* (Film). (Provo, UT: Brigham Young University, 1971).
4. Kenneth H. Cooper, *The Aerobics Way* (New York: M. Evans and Company, 1977), p. 10.
5. National Vital Statistics Division, Center for Health Statistics, Rockville, MD, 1988.
6. American College of Sports Medicine 1990: Position Stand, "The Recommended Quality and Quantity of Exercise for Developing and Maintaining Cardiorespiratory and Muscular Fitness in Healthy Adults," *Med. Sci. Sports Exerc.*, 22:2 (1990), pp. 265–274.
7. Cooper, *Run Dick, Run Jane*.
8. Lenore R. Zohman, et al., *The Cardiologists' Guide to Fitness and Health through Exercise* (New York: Simon and Schuster, 1979), p. 72.
9. *Harvard Medical School Health Letter*, 10:6 (April 1985), p. 3.
10. Ibid.
11. Ibid.
12. ACSM Position Stand, 1990.
13. Ibid.
14. Ibid.
15. Ibid.
16. Ibid.
17. Unpublished research data by Karen S. Mazzeo collected on students enrolled in aerobic dance courses, 1984-1986.
18. G. A. V. Borg, "Psychophysical Bases of Perceived Exertion." *Medicine and Science in Sport and Exercise* 14(1982). Also, Karen S. Mazzeo, *Aerobics, The Way To Fitness* (Englewood, CO: Morton Publishing Company, 1992), p. 18.
19. Charlotte A. Williams, "THR Versus RPE. The debate over monitoring exercise intensity." *IDEA Today*, April 1991, p. 42.
20. Williams, p. 42.
21. Kenneth H. Cooper, *Running Without Fear* (New York: M. Evans and Company, 1985), p. 128.
22. Ibid, p. 192.
23. Ibid, p. 197.

24. Kenneth H. Cooper, *The Aerobics Program for Total Well Being* (New York: M. Evans and Company, 1982), p. 141.

25. Lenore R. Zohman et al., *The Cardiologists' Guide to Fitness and Health Through Exercise* (New York: Simon and Schuster, 1979), p. 87.

Chapter 2

1. Joan Price, "Stepping Basics," *IDEA Today,* November/December 1990, p. 57.

2. Len Kravitz, "The Safe Way To Step," *IDEA Today,* April 1991, pp. 47–50.

3. Sports Step, Inc., videotape accompanying The Step,™ *Introduction To Step Training* (Atlanta: Sports Step, 1989).

4. Lynne Brick and David Essel, videotape, *Pump N' Step* (1991).

5. Lorna Francis, Peter Francis, and Gin Miller, *Step-Reebok. The First Aerobic Training Workout with Muscle. Instructor Training Manual* (Reebok International Ltd., 1990).

6. Ibid, p. 6.

7. M. S. Olson, et al., "Cardiorespiratory Responses to 'Aerobic' Bench Stepping Exercise in Females," *Medicine and Science in Sports and Exercise* (abstract), 23:4 (April 1991), S27.

8. D. L. Blessing, et al., "The Energy Cost of Bench Stepping With and Without One and Two Pound Hand-Held Weights," *Medicine and Science in Sports and Exercise* (abstract), 23:4 (April 1991), S28.

9. F. Goss, et al., "Energy Cost of Bench Stepping and Pumping Light Handweights in Trained Subjects," *Research Quarterly for Exercise and Sport,* 60:4 (1989), pp. 369–372.

10. L. Calarco, et al., "The Metabolic Cost of Six Common Movement Patterns of Bench Step Aerobic Dance," *Medicine and Science in Sports and Exercise* (abstract), 23:4 (April 1991), S140.

11. Ralph La Forge, "What the Latest Research Has to Say About STEP Exercise," *IDEA Today,* September 1991, pp. 31–35.

12. D. Stanforth, et al., "The Effect of Bench Height and Rate of Stepping on the Metabolic Cost of Bench Stepping," *Medicine and Science in Sports and Exercise* (abstract), 23:(4) (April 1991), S143.

13. Ibid.

14. Calcarco, et al.

15. Len Kravitz and Rich Deivert, "The Safe Way to Step," *IDEA Today,* April 1991, pp. 47–50.

16. Francis, p. 20.

17. Monica Turner, "Aerobics Step Training," *American Fitness Quarterly,* October 1990, p. 19.

18. Francis, p. 20.

19. Kravitz, et al., p. 48.

Chapter 3

1. Candice Copeland-Brooks, *Moves...and More!* (videotape) (San Diego, CA: IDEA, Inc., 1990).

2. Candice Copeland, *The Low-Impact Challenge for the Fitness Professional* (videotape) (Newark, NJ: PPI Entertainment Group/Parade Video, 1991).

3. Julie Moo-Bradley and Jerrie Moo-Thurman, *Aerobics Choreography in Action: The High-Low Impact Advantage* (videotape). (San Diego, CA: IDEA, Inc. 1990).

4. Lynne Brick, *Total Body Workout* videotape, (Philadelphia: Creative Instructors Aerobics, 1991).

5. Amy Jones, "Point-Counterpoint. Sequencing a Dance-Exercise Class," *Dance Exercise Today,* May/June 1985.

6. Lorna Francis, Peter Francis, and Gin Miller, *Step-Reebok. The First Aerobic Training Workout With Muscle. Instructor Training Manual.* (Reebok International Ltd., 1990), p. 23.

7. Len Kravitz et al., "Static and PNF Stretches," *IDEA Today,* March 1990.

8. Ibid.

9. Ibid.

10. Ibid.

Chapter 4

1. Karen S. Mazzeo, *Aerobics — The Way To Fitness* (Englewood, CO: Morton Publishing Company, 1992), pp. 95–104.

2. Lorna Francis, Peter Francis, and Gin Miller, *Step-Reebok. The First Aerobic Training Workout With Muscle. Instructor Training Manual.* (Reebok International Ltd., 1990), p. 25.
3. Ibid, p. 25.
4. Candice Copeland-Brooks, *Moves...and More!* (videotape) (San Diego: IDEA, Inc., 1990).

Chapter 5

1. *Webster's New Twentieth Century Dictionary Unabridged,* 2d ed. (New York: Simon and Schuster, 1983), p. 319.
2. Candice Copeland-Brooks, "Smooth Moves," *IDEA Today,* June 1991, p. 34.
3. Lorna Francis, Peter Francis, and Gin Miller, *Step-Reebok. The First Aerobic Training Workout With Muscle. Instructor Training Manual.* (Reebok International Ltd., 1990), p. 26.
4. Copeland-Brooks, p. 34.
5. Cathe Friedrich, *STEP "N" Motion Training Seminar,* Student Recreation Center, Bowling Green State University, Bowling Green, OH, February 1992.
6. Tamilee Webb, "Step 'Q' Signs," IDEA Fitness Renaissance Educational Conference and Fitness Expo, Pittsburgh, PA, 1991.
7. Ibid.
8. Lynn Brick, "Step I.T.," IDEA Fitness Renaissance Educational Conference and Fitness Expo, Pittsburgh, PA, 1991.

Chapter 6

1. Lorna Francis, Peter Francis, and Gin Miller, *Step-Reebok. The First Aerobic Training Workout with Muscle. Instructor Training Manual.* (Reebok International Ltd., 1990).
2. Joan Price, "Stepping Basics," *IDEA Today,* November/December 1990, p. 57.
3. Ibid.
4. Francis, p. 17.
5. Ralph La Forge, "What the Latest Research Has to Say About Step Exercise," *IDEA Today,* September 1991, p. 33.
6. L. Calarco et al., "The Metabolic Cost of Six Common Movement Patterns of Bench Step Aerobic Dance," *Medicine and Science in Sports and Exercise* (abstract), 23:4 (April 1991), S140.
7. Gin Miller, "Taking the Right Step," *IDEA Today,* October 1991, pp. 36–39.
8. Reebok Newsletter, *In Step,* Spring 1992, p. 10.
9. Greg Niederlander, *Step Strength* (videotape), (Buffalo Grove, IL: SPRI Products & Brick Bodies, 1991).
10. American College of Sports Medicine 1990: Position Stand, "The Recommended Quality and Quantity of Exercise for Developing and Maintaining Cardiorespiratory and Muscular Fitness in Healthy Adults," *Med. Sci. Sports Exercise* 22:2 (1990), pp. 265–274.
11. Sports Step, Inc., videotape accompanying The Step, *Introduction to Step Training* (Atlanta: Sports Step, 1989).
12. James L. Hesson, *Weight Training For Life* (Englewood, CO: Morton Publishing Company, 1985), Appendices pp. 164–165.
13. Karen S. Mazzeo, *Aerobics — The Way To Fitness* (Englewood, CO: Morton Publishing Co., 1992), p. 51.
14.. SPRI Products, Inc., *Pumping Rubber* (instructions for product use) SPRI, 1554 Barclay Blvd., Buffalo Grove, IL 60089, 1988.
15. Ibid.
16. Ibid.
17. American College of Obstetricians and Gynecologists, *Safety Guidelines for Women Who Exercise* (ACOG Home Exercise Programs) (Washington, DC, ACOG, 1986), p. 6.
18. Hesson, p. 33.
19. Ibid.
20. Lynn Brick, "Step I.T.," IDEA Fitness Renaissance Educational Conference and Fitness Expo, Pittsburgh, PA, 1991.
21. John Patrick O'Shea, *Scientific Principles and Methods of Strength Fitness,* 2d ed. (Reading, MA: Addison-Wesley Publishing Company, 1976), p. 89.
22. Diane Chapman, "Two-Stepping Takes Off," *IDEA Today* (Industry News), September 1992, p. 11.
23. Ibid.

Chapter 7

1. Shad Helmstetter, *What To Say When You Talk To Yourself* (New York: Pocket Books, Simon & Schuster, 1986), pp. 62–71.
2. Hugh Prather, *there is a place where you are not alone* (New York: Doubleday and Company, 1980), p. 96.
3. Anthony Robbins, *Unlimited Power* (New York: Fawcett/Columbine, 1986), p. 155.
4. Suzy Prudden, "Affirmations Work!" *IDEA Today,* April 1991, p. 57.
5. Robbins, p. 31.
6. Hans Selye, *Stress Without Distress* (Toronto: McClelland and Stewart Ltd., 1974), p. 141.
7. Roman G. Carek, Director of the Counseling and Career Development Center, Bowling Green State University, Bowling Green, Ohio, from his Stress Management presentation in the LIFE Seminar Workshop Series, 1982, held at the Student Recreation Center of BGSU.
8. Nutrition Education Services/Oregon Dairy Council, *"Super Four, A Star-Studded Guide to Food Choices"* (Portland: NES/ODC, 1991).
9. Judy Tillapaugh, "Cross-Training in the Kitchen," *IDEA Today,* October 1991, p. 21.
10. U.S. Department of Agriculture, *Food Guide Pyramid, A Guide to Daily Food Choices* (Washington, DC: U.S. Government Printing Office, 1992).
11. National Dairy Council, *Guide to Good Eating: A Recommended Daily Pattern* 4th edition (B 164-5) (Rosemont, IL: National Dairy Council, 1980). A revised pamphlet visual is available, *Guide to Good Eating,* 5th edition (0001N3) (Rosemont, IL: National Dairy Council, 1991).
12. Inservice seminar for Health Education Division Faculty of School of Health, Physical Education, and Recreation, Bowling Green State University. Bowling Green, Ohio, December, 1990, given by nutrition education consultant Jan Meyer of Dairy and Nutrition Council, Mid East, Toledo, OH.
13. Nutrition Education Services/Oregon Dairy Council, *Super Four* pamphlet.
14. National Dairy Council, *Guide to Wise Food Choices* B 170-1 (Rosemont, IL: National Dairy Council, 1978, p. 4).
15. Wholesome and Hearty Foods, Inc., "Product Line Nutritional Information," given by restaurateur Meredith 'Chip' Myles, Bowling Green, Ohio, spring 1992.
16. Nutrition Education Services/Oregon Dairy Council, *Super Four* pamphlet.
17. U.S. Department of Agriculture, Health and Human Services, Nutrition and Your Health, Dietary Guidelines for Americans, 3d edition (Home and Garden Bulletin No. 232) (Washington, DC: U.S. Government Printing Office, 1990).
18. Lucy M. Williams, lecture and literature, "Shopping Tips For Low Fat, Low Salt, Low Cholesterol Diets," delivered to Karen S. Mazzeo's Anchor Fitness-Personal Excellence® class, February, 1991.
19. Ibid.
20. U.S. Department of Agriculture, "Nutrition and Your Health, 1990.
21. Jan Lewis, *Nutrition Notes. Dietary Guidelines* 2, (Bowling Green, OH: Bowling Green State University, 1981).
22. Dr. Steven Blair, keynote speaker to the 1992 American Alliance for Health, Physical Education, Recreation & Dance National Convention, Indianapolis, IN.
23. Connirae Andreas, and Steven A. Andreas, *Heart of the Mind* (Moab, UT: Real People Press, 1989), p. 251.
24. Ibid, p. 125.
25. Lewis, p. 6.
26. Kenneth H. Cooper, *The Aerobics Way* (New York: M. Evans and Company, 1977), p. 142.
27. Lewis, p. 4.
28. Ibid.
29. Ibid.

Chapter 8

1. Anthony Robbins, *Personal Power* (audiotape series) (Irwindale, CA: Robbins Research International, Guthy-Ranker Corp., 1989).

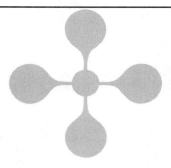

Index

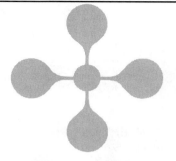

ACKNOWLEDGMENTS

Special appreciation is extended to the following individuals who have shared their time and superior talents in this endeavor:

Stephen I. Block
Richard W. Bowers, Ph.D.
Philip H. Goldstein
Jeffrey Hall
Peter Holmes
Ruth Horton
Virnette D. House
Marian Larkin
Lisa Mark

Mary Beth Mazzeo
Douglas N. Morton
Terry W. Parsons, Ph.D.
Peggy Paul, R.D., L.D.
Bernard Rabin, Ed.D.
Carrie A. Robinson
Joanne R. Saliger
Sue Schoonover
Vivian L. Smallwood

Appreciation goes to the following for granting permission to use copyrighted materials:

Kenneth Cooper, M.D., M.P.H., and Bantam/Doubleday/Dell
The National Dairy Council and The Oregon Dairy Council

A special thank you to the following companies for providing apparel and equipment with which to photograph:

Nike, Inc., One Bowerman Drive, Beaverton OR 97005
(1-800-535-6453) for women's fitness apparel

Mark Cooksey, Manager, Foot Locker — Bowling Green Mall (Ohio)
(419-354-0567) for Nike and Reebok Cross-Trainer Shoes

Sports Step, Inc., for The Steps and instructional videos. For additional information on The Step™, call Sports Step, Inc. (1-800-SAY STEP)

SPRI Products, Inc., 1554 Barclay Blvd., Buffalo Grove, IL 60089
(1-800-222-7774) for men's tee-shirts, rubber resistance bands and tubing

To all the people who have supported and inspired me in striving to reach my goals, especially

- Michael, Nicholas, and Anthony with love and appreciation of what is really important in life

- Raymond and Marilynn for their love, guidance, and encouragement to pursue my interests

- Andy and Louise for their love and assistance in allowing me to take part in this exciting experience

Thanks to all who have encouraged me to not just dream about my goals but have helped make them happen.

Lauren

To Dr. Lee A. Meserve, a "Master Teacher" in every sense of the word — role model of personal fitness excellence, compassionate friend, and teacher willing to share his talents and expertise regarding the human condition, to those like myself who are eager to learn.

And to Dr. Bernie Rabin, a role model of physical fitness and mental training excellence whose expertise in peak performance initially sparked and continues to fuel my interest in tapping into one's unlimited potential.

Karen